Anaesthesiology and Resuscitation
Anaesthesiologie und Wiederbelebung
Anesthésiologie et Réanimation

57

Editors

Prof. Dr. R. Frey, Mainz · Dr. F. Kern, St. Gallen
Prof. Dr. O. Mayrhofer, Wien

Managing Editor: Prof. Dr. M. Halmágyi, Mainz

Das Ultrakurznarkoticum Methohexital

*Bericht über das Internationale Methohexital-Symposion
am 5. Dezember 1970 in Frankfurt/M.*

Herausgegeben von

Charlotte Lehmann

Mit 55 Abbildungen

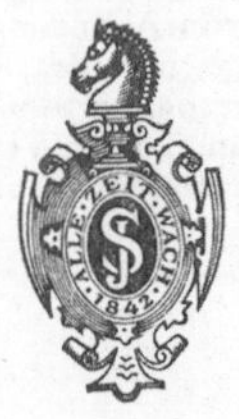

Springer-Verlag Berlin Heidelberg New York 1972

ISBN-13: 978-3-540-05576-1   e-ISBN-13: 978-3-642-46276-4
DOI: 10.1007/978-3-642-46276-4

Vorwort

Die in diesem Band enthaltenen Referate und Diskussionsbemerkungen
stellen einen vollständigen Bericht über die am 5. 12. 1970 in Frankfurt/
Main stattgefundene Tagung dar. Vor 150 Anaesthesiologen berichteten
Wissenschaftler und Kliniker aus England, Frankreich und Deutschland
sowohl über die pharmakologischen und physiologischen Grundlagen als
auch über die klinische Anwendung des Methohexitals, eines methylierten
Oxybarbiturates.

Dieses Ultrakurznarkoticum, das 1954 bei ELI LILLY in Indianapolis
entwickelt und 1960 eingeführt wurde, fand zunächst fast ausschließlich in
seinem Heimatland Verwendung. In Deutschland bürgerte sich sein Gebrauch nur zögernd ein, weil rührigere Arzneimittelbetriebe ausreichend
viele ähnliche Präparate vertrieben.

Erst die erneute und intensive Suche nach einem Ultrakurznarkoticum,
das sowohl die bisher geforderten Voraussetzungen wie schnellen Wirkungseintritt und kurze Erholungsphase, also rasch wiederhergestellte Straßenfähigkeit aufweist, als auch das Risiko exzessiver Histaminfreisetzung vermeiden läßt, verhalf dem Präparat zum Durchbruch.

Eine während der Diskussion gestellte und wegen der Aussagekraft
derartiger Angaben durchaus berechtigte Frage, wieviel Ampullen die
Firma bisher verkauft habe, wieviel Narkosen also in etwa durchgeführt
wurden, kann jetzt beantwortet werden. Das Werk teilte mit, daß in den
Jahren von 1960 bis 1970 7027 kg Trockensubstanz Absatz fanden. Wenn
man als durchschnittlich verwendete Menge 150 mg ansetzt, läßt sich behaupten, daß bisher also etwa 47 Millionen Anaesthesien durchgeführt
wurden. Damit kann gesagt werden, daß Methohexital durchaus er-
probt ist.

Der Herausgeber dankt Herrn Professor FREY, der das Präparat in
Deutschland als erster anwendete, sich also traditionelle Verdienste erwarb,
für die Übernahme des Vorsitzes und den Referenten und Diskussionsteil-
nehmern für ihre interessanten Beiträge, die das Gelingen dieser Tagung
sicherten.

München, Januar 1972 CH. LEHMANN

Inhaltsverzeichnis

Verzeichnis der Referenten

BAUER-EHNES, HANNELORE, Dr. med., Anaesthesie-Abteilung der Chirurgischen Klinik und Poliklinik am Klinikum rechts der Isar der Technischen Universität München

BEER, R., Prof. Dr. med., Vorstand des Institutes für Anaesthesiologie an der Chirurgischen Universitätsklinik München

BUXTON, J. D., M. D., New Cross Hospital, London, England

CHLADEK, F., Dr. med., Anaesthesie-Abteilung am Zentral-Krankenhaus Links der Weser, Bremen

COLEMAN, D. J., M. D., St. George's Hospital, London, England

DARBOVEN, OLIVA, Dr. med., Anaesthesie-Abteilung der Chirurgischen Klinik und Poliklinik am Klinikum rechts der Isar der Technischen Universität München

ELCHLEPP, F., Dr. med., Anaesthesie-Abteilung der Chirurgischen Klinik und Poliklinik am Klinikum rechts der Isar der Technischen Universität München

FINK, CHRISTA, Dr. med., Anaesthesie-Abteilung der Chirurgischen Klinik und Poliklinik am Klinikum rechts der Isar der Technischen Universität München

FREY, R., Prof. Dr. med., Direktor des Instituts für Anaesthesiologie der Universität Mainz

GAUTHIER-LAFAYE, J. P., Prof. Dr. med., Département d'Anesthésiologie, Strasbourg, France

GROSS, G., Dr. med., Anaesthesie-Abteilung am St. Elisabeth-Krankenhaus Köln-Hohenlind

HARTUNG, ANGELA, Dr. med., Anaesthesie-Abteilung der Chirurgischen Klinik und Poliklinik am Klinikum rechts der Isar der Technischen Universität München

KAY, B., M. D., Derbyshire Children's Hospital, Derby, England

LANDAUER, B., Dr. med., Anaesthesie-Abteilung der Chirurgischen Klinik und Poliklinik am Klinikum rechts der Isar der Technischen Universität München

LANDAUER, GABY, Dr. med., Anaesthesie-Abteilung der Chirurgischen Klinik und Poliklinik am Klinikum rechts der Isar der Technischen Universität München

LEHMANN, CHARLOTTE, Dr. med., Chefarzt der Anaesthesie-Abteilung der Chirurgischen Klinik und Poliklinik am Klinikum rechts der Isar der Technischen Universität München

MEIER, CHRISTA, Dr. med., Anaesthesie-Abteilung der Chirurgischen Klinik und Poliklinik am Klinikum rechts der Isar der Technischen Universität München

ROGGENKÄMPER, RENATE, Dr. med., Anaesthesie-Abteilung der Chirurgischen Klinik und Poliklinik am Klinikum rechts der Isar der Technischen Universität München

RUDOLPH, P., Dr. med., Abteilung für Anaesthesiologie der Universität Würzburg

SOGA, DUBRAVKA, Priv.-Doz. Dr. med., Institut für Anaesthesiologie an der Chirurgischen Universitätsklinik München

STOFFREGEN, J., Prof. Dr. med., Direktor des Instituts für Klinische Anaesthesie der Universität Göttingen

WEBER, K., Dr. med., Chefarzt der Anaesthesie-Abteilung am St. Elisabeth-Krankenhaus Köln-Hohenlind

WHITWAM, J. G., M. D., Hammersmith Hospital, London, England

WILCKENS, INGRID, Dr. med., Anaesthesie-Abteilung der Chirurgischen Klinik und Poliklinik am Klinikum rechts der Isar der Technischen Universität München

Eröffnung

Von **Rudolf Frey**

In den letzten 30 Jahren sind über ein Dutzend intravenöse Kurznarkotica entwickelt worden, teils Barbiturate, teils Thiobarbiturate, teils Eugenolderivate. Ihre Vor- und Nachteile gegeneinander abzuwägen ist das Ziel unseres heutigen Symposions.

Das Methohexital ist eine ganz besondere Substanz: Es ist ein Barbiturat (nicht ein Thiobarbiturat), also etwas weniger toxisch für das Herz, und sehr viel stärker wirksam als alle anderen Barbiturate, die wir bisher gekannt haben.

Im deutschen Schrifttum wurden relativ wenige Arbeiten über das Methohexital veröffentlicht; es ist zu wenig darüber bekannt, obwohl bis heute insgesamt an die 50 Millionen Anaesthesien mit diesem Mittel durchgeführt worden sind.

Um so dankbarer bin ich, daß einige Experten, die sich seit Jahren intensiv mit dieser Substanz befassen – sowohl mit der pharmakologischen Grundlagenforschung als auch mit der klinischen Anwendung – und die über tausende oder zehntausende von persönlichen Erfahrungen verfügen, uns heute hierüber berichten werden, so daß wir am Schluß des Symposions ein klares Bild über die Einordnung des Methohexital in unseren Arzneischatz haben werden.

Damit eröffne ich unser Symposion und bitte nun als ersten Redner Mr. WHITWAM aus London.

The Pharmacology of Brietal Sodium (Methohexitone Sodium)

By **J. G. Whitwam**

Department of Anaesthetics,
The Royal Postgraduate Medical School, London W. 12, England

The drug in this discussion "Brietal Sodium" will be referred to by its B. P. name i. e. methohexitone sodium. This drug was introduced because of the need for an anaesthetic agent which had a shorter duration of action, less cumulative effect, fewer undesirable side effexts e. g. cardiovascular depression, respiratory depression, local irritation of the tissues, and which would also provide better reflex depression at a lighter level of narcosis than existing intravenous induction agents. Because so much of the literature about anaesthetic agents compares the effects of various drugs, it is inevitable that in describing the pharmacological properties of methohexitone some reference will be made to other drugs of similar purpose. For example thiopentone, described by TABERN and VOLWILER in 1935, was first used in clinical anaesthesia thirty six years ago; the experience with this agent is so wide, and such is its reliability and consistency of effect, that it provides a standard against which newer drugs can be assessed.

Structure

BARRON and DUNDEE (1961) compared the structural formulae of many of the barbiturates which have been used as agents for induction of anaesthesia including methohexitone. In general, substitution of oxygen for sulphur in position 2 in the barbiturate nucleus produces a drug which has a shorter duration of action while modification of the side chains at position 5, in an attempt to shorten the duration of action may produce a drug which has excitatory or convulsive properties.

The pharmacology of the barbiturate 1 methyl - 5 (1 methyl - 2 pentynyl -) 5 allyl-barbituric acid was first reported by GIBSON et al. in 1955. When introduced, this drug represented a departure from the conventional barbiturate anaesthetics because it contains no sulphur atom, has both acetylinic and olefinic unsaturations in the 5 position radicals and contains a methyl group on one of the ring nitrogens. The structural formula is shown in Fig. 1.

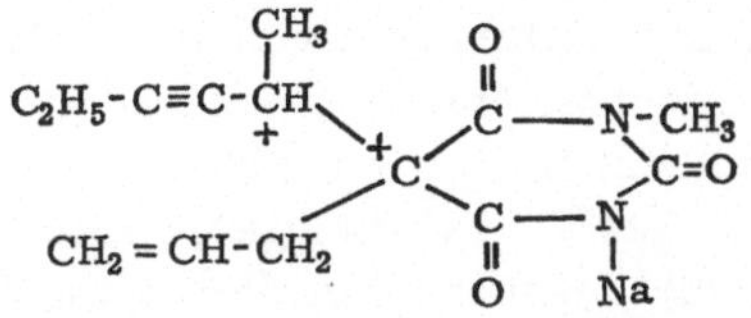

Fig. 1. Structural formula of methohexitone (sodium d1-1 methyl-5-(methyl-2-pentynyl)-5-allyl-barbituric acid). + denotes positions of asymetry

There are two asymetric carbon atoms and hence four stereoisomers are possible. Dextro- and Laevo- (d and l) forms exist as a result of a change in configuration about the asymetric carbon atom of the pentynyl radical; α and β forms occur due to the asymetric C-5 atom of the barbiturate ring. Thus there are two racemic mixtures α dl and β dl. GIBSON *et al.* (1959) described the pharmacological properties of all four stereoisomers. The β dl mixture was found to be approximately 50% more potent than α dl, but also produced a higher incidence of undesirable stimulant effects.

The drug which was originally introduced to clinical practice was a mixture of α dl and β dl stereoisomers (compound 22451) and was first used in electroconvulsive therapy (CHERNISH *et al.*, 1956). The rapid onset of anaesthesia and the subsequent rapid recovery was confirmed by GRUBER *et al.* (1956). However, the incidence of excitatory side effects was unacceptably high (GRUBER *et al.*, 1957) and the clinical trial of 22451 was abandoned.

In 1957 STOELTING described the pharmacology and early clinical experience of the α dl isomer (compound 25398) which has a higher melting point than the β dl isomer. The α dl isomer was found to have a high potency and was associated with rapid recovery from anaesthesia and a low incidence of side effects. This substance is known as brietal sodium, methohexitone sodium (B.P.) and sodium methohexital (U.S.N.F.)

Administration

Methohexitone sodium (Brietal sodium) is presented as a white crystalline powder mixed with anhydrous sodium carbonate (6% by weight), and may be dissolved in water, 5% dextrose or saline. The pH limits of a 5% solution in carbon dioxide free water are 11.1 to 11.4 (B.P.) and mixing with acid solutions such as atropine sulphate, tubocurarine and suxamethonium is not to be recommended. Although it is usually administered intravenously it may be given intramuscularly or rectally. Oral use has been tried and found to be unsatisfactory (COLEMAN and GREEN, 1960).

Uptake and Distribution

In 1960 Price described the kinetics of the distribution of thiopentone in the body and other barbiturates have a qualitatively similar pattern of distribution. In the first phase, thiopentone added to the blood forms a "central pool", and the amount of drug in the blood is lost rapidly, primarily as a result of uptake by the perfused viscera (heart, kidney, splanchnic area, and central nervous system) so that at 1 min, 55% of the drug is present in these tissues even though they represent only 6% of body weight. Thus following the administration of a single intravenous dose of a barbiturate, the peak concentration in the brain will occur after 1 min, and it has been shown by electroencephalography that the maximum effect of the drug on the central nervous system also occurs at this time (Price et al., 1957). During the second phase, the drug is redistributed from rapidly perfused viscera, including the brain, to the lean body mass such as muscle and skin, so that after 5 min the maximal concentration in the brain will have been reduced by half; fat uptake is insignificant at this stage. After 30 min the brain will contain only 5% of the injected dose, fat 18% and lean body mass 75% and poorly perfused tissues, e.g. ligaments, tendons and cartilage play only a small part in the redistribution of the drug. During the third phase considerable uptake of the drug by the fatty tissues occurs so that, 2–3 hrs after injection, the concentration there exceeds that of other tissues. Full redistribution takes 8–10 hrs at which time metabolic degradation has reduced the total amount of drug in the body to less than 20% of the administered dose.

It seems likely that methohexitone will be similar to thiopentone in its pattern of distribution immediately after injection. However, methohexitone has a smaller oil to water portion ratio than thiopentone and is less extensively localised in fat (Brand et al., 1963), so that there are quantitative differences in the distribution of the two drugs.

Recovery of consciousness after a single intravenous dose of either thiopentone or methohexitone is caused largely by redistribution of the drug into lean body mass, which explains why the small muscular individual often requires a larger dose of drug, on a weight basis, than a heavier obese person. This is also one factor in the larger doses required for men as compared with women who have a lower ratio of muscle to fat than men (Young and Whitwam, 1964). However, an increase in body weight from whatever cause will in general increase drug requirement.

Blood Levels

In 1966 Sunshine and his associates studied aortic and venous blood levels of methohexitone in human subjects following single intravenous injections of 1.5 mg/kg to 2 mg/kg given as a 1% solution in a time of 10–15 sec. Maximal aortic blood levels occurred within the first minute and, reached a maximum concentration of 7.2 mg/ per 100 ml, of blood when 2 mg/kg was administered in 10 sec. At 2 min, the blood levels fell to between 0.5 mg% and 0.8 mg% while at 5 min the recorded values were between 0.21 mg% and 0.29 mg%. The drug was not demonstrated in blood drawn from the median antecubital vein in the arm not used for injection of the drug earlier than 1 min from the time of injection. The highest value observed in venous blood was 1.7 mg% and occurred within the first 90 sec, which in view of the aortic blood levels obtained during a similar period, shows the rapid distribution of the drug into the tissues of the forearm.

An ionised drug such as methohexitone will not pass freely across cell membranes, and hence free distribution into the intracellular water cannot occur. In order to produce the observed fall in blood levels during the first 5 min after administration, extensive binding of the drug must occur in the body tissues, which must also be reversible to allow rapid redistribution of the drug between the various tissues.

Transport in Blood

In human plasma 73% of methohexitone was found to be bound to plasma protein (BRAND *et al.*, 1963) and in whole blood with a haematocrit of 42%, approximately 20% of the drug was also found to be in the red cell mass (WHITWAM, 1965). Thus only 7% of the drug will be free in the plasma of which 76% will be unionised (i.e. active) at pH 4,4 (BRAND *et al.*, 1963).

Thus a reduction in either plasma proteins or red cell mass will leave more drug free in an active form and this may be a factor contributing to the increased effectiveness of the drug in anaemic patients.

Uptake by Fat

BRAND *et al.* (1963) found 26 mg/kg and 51 mg/kg of methohexitone in subcutaneous fat, 1 hr and 2 hrs respectively after the administration of 1.9 g of the drug during 30 min, values for omental fat being somewhat lower. SUNSHINE *et al.* (1966) found trace amounts of methohexitone in fat 15–30 min after a single intravenous dose of 2 mg/kg, and 3 hrs after such a dose the fat concentration reached 0.6 mg/kg; in two patients (weight 67 kg) who received 350 mg and 1 g of the drug, during 90 min, fat levels of 1.4 mg/kg and 5 mg/kg were found 90 min after completing the infusion of methohexitone. The maximum value in fat (5 mg/kg) reported by SUN-SHINE *et al.* (1966) 90 min after infusion of 1 g of the drug is only 10% of the value (51 mg/kg) found by BRAND *et al.* (1963) 95 min after completing an infusion of 1.9 g in 30 min. The differences between the two studies may be due to differences in the rate of infusion, the larger amount of drug used by BRAND and his associates, differences in the ratio of lean body mass to fat in the very small number of patients studied, and the greater specificity of gaschromatography (SUNSHINE *et al.*, 1966) as compared with the ultraviolet absorption method used by BRAND *et al.* (1963).

Passage into Brain

BRAND *et al.* (1963) recorded the EEG during intravenous injection of methohexitone and concluded that the drug passes rapidly from blood to brain as is the case with thiopentone (KIERSEY *et al.*, 1952; PRICE *et al.*, 1957).

Placental Transmission

MARSHALL (1964) showed that methohexitone, like other barbiturates crosses the placenta. However, there was no significant respiratory depression observed in infants whose mothers had received methohexitone in doses ranging from 85 mg to 120 mg.

Metabolism and Excretion

Barbiturates are metabolised in the liver (McMAHON, 1963) and produce depression of liver function, although methohexitone produces less depression than thiopentone when administered in equipotent anaesthetic doses (BITTRICH *et al.*, 1963).

WELLES *et al.* (1963) studied the metabolism and excretion of methohexitone in the rat and the dog. They found no unchanged drug in the urine, but using paper chromatography found evidence for the existence of several metabolites in the urine, the most abundant of which they succeeded in identifying as 1 methyl-5-ally-5- (1 methyl-4 hydroxy-2 pentynyl) barbituric acid formed by hydroxylation of the penultimate carbon of the pentynyl side chain. Demethylation of the N-methyl group did not occur to a great extent so that in a 7 hr period after administration of N-methyl labelled methohexitone (C^{14}) only 0.54% and 1.40% of the radioactivity was recovered as $C^{14}O_2$ in the expired air of the rat and the dog respectively. Excretion of metabolites was very rapid. In the rat 50% of the radioactivity of a C^{14} labelled dose of drug appeared in the bile in 1 h, which increased to 70% within 3 hrs, and the total faecal excretion of metabolites was 82.7%. The dog excreted by both urinary and biliary routes amounting to 21.7% of the radioactivity of a labelled dose in the first hour and 52.4% in 8 hrs. Total faecal excretion in the dog was 30.1%.

SUNSHINE *et al.* (1966) found trace amounts of methohexitone in urine and bile of human subjects who received up to 1.0 g of the drug. In extracts from urine consistent evidence for the existence of two metabolites was obtained, but identification was not possible. Less than 1% of the administered dose was excreted as unchanged methohexitone.

Rate of Biotransformation

WELLES *et al.* (1963) found in the dog, that after an initial phase, when the blood level of methohexitone fell rapidly from 10–20 min (measured as radioactivity after administration of C^{14} labelled drug), the rate of disappearance of radioactivity from the blood from 30 min to 6 hrs after administration was 24.6% per hour. This is in approximate agreement with BRAND *et al.* (1963) who found in man that after a large loading dose, the rate of decrease of the concentration of methohexitone in blood was 15–19% per hour.

Clinical Pharmacology

Potency

Methohexitone is among the most potent intravenous induction agents and is approximately three times as potent as thiopentone (e.g. REDISH *et al.*, 1958; BELLVILLE *et al.*, 1960; GREEN and JOLLY, 1960; CLARKE *et al.*, 1968). HOWELLS *et al.* (1967) reported that methohexitone was 5.2 times as potent as propanidid. However, CLARKE *et al.* (1968) produced a lower ratio of 1 to 3.63.

Intravenous Administration

1. Induction of Anaesthesia

Probably the best approach to a discussion of the induction characteristics of an agent is that introduced by Professor DUNDEE and his collegues (DUNDEE and RIDING, 1960; DUNDEE *et al.*, 1960; DUNDEE and MOORE, 1961).

Induction complications are classified as follows.

a) Excitatory phenomena i.e. tremors and involuntary muscle movements mostly involving the limbs.
b) Respiratory upset i.e. cough, hiccough or laryngospasm.
c) Respiratory depression.
d) Cardiovascular changes.

A. Excitatory Phenomena. Muscle movements and tremors were not reported in original observations of STOELTING (1957), but TAYLOR and STOELTING (1960) reported a 3% incidence. Since then the incidence of these complications has varied from very low to as high as 35–40% in various reports, depending on dose, premedication and other factors (e.g. REDISH *et al.*, 1958; WYANT and CHANG, 1959; DUNDEE and MOORE, 1961a and b, MOORE and DUNDEE, 1961; WHITWAM and MANNERS, 1962). These complications are rarely troublesome, and quickly disappear.

B. Respiratory Upset. Here again the incidence of cough, hiccough and laryngospasm varies in different reports and can be as high as 40 to 45%

(MOORE and DUNDEE, 1961; YOUNG and WHITWAM, 1964a). Laryngospasm when it occurs while the patient is mainly under the influence of methohexitone is usually mild and passes off rapidly (TAYLOR and STOELTING, 1960; YOUNG and WHITWAM, 1964).

Factors Influencing Excitatory Phenomena and Respiratory Upset

DUNDEE and his associates (1961) showed that the following factors will influence the appearance of these side effects.

1. The dose of methohexitone — larger doses will produce a higher incidence of complications. YOUNG and WHITWAM (1964a) also provided data showing the increased incidence of side effects as the dose of methohexitone is increased.

2. Strength of solution. 2% solution was found to give a higher incidence of side effects than 1% solution. WYANT et al. (1957) also found a higher incidence of side effects when the drug was used as a 2.5% solution as compared with 1% which is presumably due to the faster injection of drug with the stronger solution.

3. Preanaesthetic medication. Hyoscine causes a higher incidence than atropine. Drugs which increase the sensitivity to tibial pain cause a high incidence of complications and in this respect promethazine is one of the worst offenders. Drugs with analgesic properties, e.g. pethidine, lower the incidence of complications.

Thus in order to minimise the incidence of these complications, premedication should be restricted to atropine and an analgesic drug e.g. pethidine or opiate, while methohexitone should be administered slowly as a 1% solution in small doses.

TAYLOR and STOELTING (1960) considered methohexitone suitable for asthmatic patients. The respiratory complications sometimes associated with the use of methohexitone are transient, and it is not contra-indicated in patients with chest disease.

C. Respiratory depression. There have been conflicting reports on the effects of methohexitone on respiration. WEYL et al. (1958) reported a very low incidence of respiratory depression, and COLEMAN and GREEN (1960) reviewing 10,142 administrations of methohexitone commented on the absence of apnoea, which was confirmed by JOLLY (1960) and GREEN and JOLLY (1960). However TAYLOR and STOELTING (1960) described the administration of methohexitone in 3,340 patients premedicated with opiate and atropine or hyoscine. They observed that respiratory depression was a frequent occurrence and apnoea occurred in 569 patients, lasting up to three minutes. WYANT and CHANG (1959) stated that whereas apnoea with thiopentone was a fairly constant phenomenon it was less consistently seen after methohexitone but tended to be a good deal more prolonged when it did occur.

WHITWAM (1962) found that there was no difference in the incidence and mean duration of apnoea after equipotent doses of methohexitone and thiopentone in patients premedicated with atropine, although the standard deviation of the duration of apnoea was greater for methohexitone indicating the greater consistency of effect with thiopentone. A dose of 1.57 mg/kg of methohexitone produced apnoea in 47 out of 66 patients which had an average duration of 28 sec. COLEMAN and GREEN (1960) who reported a virtual absence of apnoea used much smaller doses (1 mg/kg).

WYANT and BARR (1960) using thiopentone 2.5% and methohexitone 1% in a double-blind study on a similar series of patients could also find no difference in the incidence and mean duration of apnoea. They concluded that the difference between the two investigations (i. e. WYANT and CHANG, 1959 and WYANT and BARR, 1960) was due to the relatively more cautions administration of the newer drug, methohexitone, compared with the more familiar thiopentone in the earlier study.

The records published by ZINDLER (1965) show that although propanidid causes initial respiratory stimulation, this may be followed by periods of apnoea lasting up to 1 min and in terms of respiratory depression this drug appears to be no better than the barbiturates.

ECKENHOFF and HELRICH (1958) showed that opiates enhance the adverse effects of thiopentone on respiration and DUNDEE et al. (1961) have shown that this is also true for methohexitone. The papers of DUNDEE and MOORE (1961) and MOORE and DUNDEE (1961) suggest that the effect of opiate premedication on the appearance of marked respiratory depression immediately following induction of anaesthesia is greater in the case of methohexitone than with thiopentone.

Thus the occurrence of respiratory depression and the incidence of apnoea after the injection of methohexitone will depend on preanesthetic medication, and the dose and rate of administration of the drug.

D. Cardiovascular Depression. The drugs currently used for induction of anaesthesia, all produce some degree of cardiovascular depression with the exception of the phencyclidine derivative ketamine (CORRSEN and DOMINO, 1966). One of the advantages of methohexitone compared with other barbiturates is that it produces relatively less cardiovascular depression.

The clinical literature comparing the cardiovascular effects of methohexitone and thiopentone on the circulation is extensive. The original studies by WYANT et. al. (1957) and DOBKIN and WYANT (1957) concluded that the two drugs had similar effects, but that methohexitone had the disadvantage of producing hypotension. However, these studies were carried out at a time when the relative potencies of the two drugs were being assessed. For example in the study of WYANT et. al. (1957) both drugs were given as 2.5% solution, and the mean doses of thiopentone and methohexitone were 790 mg and 480 mg respectively; these would hardly be regarded as comparable doses today. Since then the clinical reports consistently refer to the smaller effect on blood pressure produced by methohexitone as compared with thiopentone (e.g. Dundee and Moore, 1961; Moore and Dundee, 1961; Whitwam and Manners, 1962).

The relative effects of methohexitone and propanidid on the circulation are not clear.

In 1965 Sankawa comparing the effects of methohexitone and propanidid in the dog stated that both drugs caused peripheral vasodilation, and that cardiac compensation was better with propanidid than methohexitone. However, their preparations had been anaesthetised for 6 h with pentobarbital before the effects of propanidid and methohexitone were studied. More recently Johnstone and Barron (1968) regarded the cardiovascular depression which follows the administration of propanidid to be cardiac in origin. In the dog Conway *et al.* (1968) found that whereas thiopentone and methohexitone caused similar reductions in arterial pressure and minor changes in cardiac output, propanidid was three times as potent in its effect on arterial pressure, and unlike the barbiturates it caused a marked increase in right ventricular pressure. Although return of the arterial pressure to control levels was rapid with all three agents, the recovery was maintained only in the case of thiopentone and methohexitone. During recovery from propanidid the pressure was maintained for four minutes, but then fell again to levels observed immediately after injection; slow recovery then occurred over the next 60 min.

The clinical position as regards the relative effects on blood pressure is not clear. Thus in 1965 Dundee suggested that equipotent doses of methohexitone caused a slightly greater deleterious cardiovascular depression than propanidid, but the doses of the two drugs – 1.6 mg/kg for methohexitone and 4 mg/kg of propanidid – represent a higher dose than would normally be used for methohexitone and a potency ratio of only 1 to 2.5. Moreover the data of Radnay (1965) would suggest that the effect of the two drugs on blood pressure was comparable. Before any definite conclusions can be reached regarding the relative effects of the two drugs on the human cardiovascular system, a further detailed study of the effects of truly equipotent doses is required.

In addition in a relatively recent paper, Woodruff *et al.* (1968) have shown that the incidence of cardiac arrythmias during electroconvulsive therapy is less in patients receiving methohexitone than in those induced with thiopentone thereby confirming the findings of Pitts *et al.* (1965).

Other Complications

Pain on injection. Taylor and Stoelting reported a high incidence of pain during injection of the drug, but subsequent papers e.g. Coleman and GREEN (1960) failed to confirm this finding. ROWLANDS (1969) found that approximately 5 % of patients felt pain during induction, but that this could be reduced to 1 % by speeding up the rate of injection of the drug. He concluded that injection pain was remembered in nearly half the patients who experienced it; the incidence of pain was the same whether the drug was dissolved in 0.9 % saline, 5 % glucose or water, and that the incidence of injection pain was almost eliminated by the addition of 1 mg of lignocaine to 10 mg of methohexitone in 1 % solution.

Arterial damage. Since the description of the sequelae of the intra-arterial injection of thiopentone by COHEN (1948), this has been an important consideration when administering any new intravenous drug. FRANCIS (1964) and MATHER and GOODHEAD (1966) found that thiopentone and methohexitone in equal amounts caused similar damage when injected intra-arterially into the rabbits ear. Since methohexitone is normally administered in only one third the dose of thiopentone, they considered methohexitone, as used in clinical practise, to be safer in this respect.

Intra-muscular administration. Methohexitone has been used intra-muscularly for induction of sleep, and is particularly suitable for children (e. g. MILLER *et al.*, 1961; MILLER and STOELTING, 1963; DRYDEN and MOSHIER 1963; RULE *et al.*, 1967). Following an adequate dose (6.6 mg/kg as a 2 % solution in normal saline), quiet onset of sleep follows within 10 min in 85 % of subjects. Complications do occur e. g. hiccough, and respiratory depression, and all authors stress the importance of continuous observation of the subject in case apnoea occurs. No serious complications at the site of injection have been reported.

Rectal Administration. Methohexitone has been administered rectally (COLEMAN and GREEN, 1960). The recommended dose is 22–33 mg/kg (maximum dose 500 mg) as a 10 % solution in tap water at room remperature in unpremedicated subjects. Sleep was induced within 5–10 min in over 80 % of subjects whose ages ranged from 5 weeks to 14 years. Apnoea occurred in 4 subjects and children under 1 year showed a 33 % incidence of induction complications.

Maintenance of Anaesthesia

GIBSON *et al.* (1955) noted that the compound 22451 had less cumulative action than either pentothal or thioseconal. CLARK and DUNDEE (1966) showed that thiopentone was more cumulative and propanidid appreciably less cumulative than methohexitone. When administered in repeated doses, or by intravenous infusion, methohexitone has been found to be suitable for use either as the sole anaesthetic agent (e. g. LISCOMBE, 1968; TEPFER, 1964; COLEMAN and DEVILLIERS, 1964) or to maintain hypnosis during surgery under local analgesia (MEAGHER, 1964 and GREEN, 1969). The level of narcosis required to produce adequate reflex depression is less than with thiopentone, so that there is no need to abolish the eyelash reflex to produce adequate anaesthesia (WHITWAM and MANNERS, 1962).

Recovery from Anaesthesia

There is little doubt that compared with thiopentone, methohexitone provides faster recovery. The awakening time following equipotent doses may be the same for the two drugs (WHITWAM and MANNERS, 1962), however, full recovery occurs more rapidly with methohexitone, and there are obvious clinical differences between the two drugs within 10–15 min of administration (e. g. EGBERT *et al.*, 1959; DUNDEE and MOORE, 1961; BARLOW and GOTTLICK, 1962; BARRY *et al.*, 1962; ELLIOT *et al.*, 1962). However, there is as yet no wholly satisfactory explanation for the observed differences between the two drugs. (BRAND *et al.*, 1963; SUNSHINE *et al.*, 1966).

When compared with propanidid the position is not as clear as with thiopentone. HOWELLS in 1967 found that awakening time after equipotent doses of methohexitone and propanidid were the same. SWERDLOW (1969) comparing the results of studies by SWERDLOW and MOORE (1967 and 1969) on propanidid and methohexitone, reached the conclusion that the time to full recovery was shorter with 0.8 mg/kg methohexitone compared with 5 mg/kg propanidid, but was much longer with 1.7 mg/kg of methohexitone compared with propanidid in a dose of 11 mg/kg. In other words using methohexitone and propanidid in a ratio of 1 to 6.5, recovery was faster with the smaller doses of methohexitone, and slower when using the larger doses. One of the problems of assessing relative recovery rates is the question of the relative potency of the drugs. CLARKE *et al.* (1968) have challenged the potency ratio of 1 of methohexitone to 5.2 of propanidid, suggesting that the latter figure should be 3.63. HANNINGTON-KIFF (1970) has measured the postoperative extraocular muscle balance (after thiopentone, methohexitone and propanidid) with a Maddox-wing. The doses administered were 1.2 mg/kg of methohexitone and 4.0 mg/kg of propanidid, i. e. a ratio of 1 to 3.3, which according to CLARKE *et al.* (1968) should load the study against methohexitone, in spite of which extraocular muscle balance recovered more quickly after methohexitone. Recovery after thiopentone (dose 3.6 mg/kg) was much slower than after propanidid and methohexitone. Recovery with all three intravenous agents was much slower than in a group of subjects who were anaesthetised with nitrous oxide, oxygen and halothane.

Post-operative Nausea and Vomiting

Barbiturate anaesthesia is associated with a low incidence of nausea and vomiting and methohexitone is no exception (YOUNG and WHITWAM, 1964;

KNAPP and BEECHER, 1956; GOLDMAN and HARRIS, 1963). Propanidid produces a much higher incidence of post anaesthetic nausea and retching (DUNDEE and CLARKE, 1964; DUNDEE, 1965; HANNINGTON-KIFF, 1970).

"Scoline Pains"

There is a lower incidence of postoperative scoline pains when methohexitone is used as the induction agent than is the case with thiopentone (CLARKE *et al.*, 1964). In this respect methohexitone and propanidid are similar.

Post Anaesthetic Vein Complications

YOUNG and WHITWAM (1964) found that in 200 patients, who had been anaesthetised with methohexitone (1 % solution) and whose veins were subsequently examined at a later date, there was not one instance of thrombosis or inflammation. HEWITT *et al.* (1966) studied the incidence of venous complications in patients who had been anaesthetised with 5 % thiopentone, 2 % methohexitone and 5 % propanidid; the latter drug produced significantly more complications than the two barbiturates.

Neuropharmacology

Electro-encephalogram (EEG)

Methohexitone resembles other barbiturates in its effects on the EEG (RIFFIN, 1960) which are similar to those of thiopentone (BELLVILLE *et al.*, 1960), and after an anaesthetic dose of methohexitone EEG changes may persist for several hours (DOENICKE and KUGLER, 1965). In the diagnostic field methohexitone is proving valuable since very small doses will cause the appearance of typical EEG activity in a large proportion of patients with suspected petit mal and temporal lobe epilepsy (GUMPERT and PAUL, 1970). Methohexitone is not contra-indicated in epileptic patients.

Action on Neurones

Recently RICHENS *et al.* (1969 a and b) showed that methohexitone impaired conduction in presynaptic terminals, long before conduction through polysynaptic pathways was blocked. Methohexitone also caused an increase in excitability of the motoneurone membrane so that while the polysynaptic component of ventral root responses was depressed, the monosynaptic component could be enhanced. Thiopentone and propanidid cause effects which are similar to those of methohexitone, while volatile agents in general block synaptic transmission and lower the excitability of the motoneurone membrane while at the same time having little effect on conduction in presynaptic terminals.

MENDELL and WALL (1964) showed that pentobarbitone abolished presynaptic hyperpolisation produced by stimulation of small afferent fibres which would have the effect of reducing the flow of afferent sensory information into the spinal cord. The work of RICHENS (1969a and b) shows that methohexitone will have a similar effects.

MENDELL and WALL (1964) showed that activity in large afferent fibres caused depolarisation of terminal afferent fibres whereas activity in small myelinated and unmyelinated (or C) fibres hyperpolarised the terminals, making entering impulses more effective. Higher centres also control the presynaptic membrane potential of afferent sensory fibres (ANDERSEN, ECCLES and SEARS, 1964; WALL, 1967). Presynaptic control of afferent sensory information forms the basis of the "Gate" control theory of pain (MELZACK and WALL, 1965).

ROBSON *et al.* (1965) showed in man that barbiturates raised the threshold of pain produced by applying heat to the skin and simultaneously lowered that produced by tibial pressure, demonstrating that the two types of pain are neurologically different; nitrous oxide and halothane increased the pain threshold for both types of stimuli and they related the difference between volatile agents and barbiturates to the influence of the latter on presynaptic conduction in the spinal cord.

It seems probable that depression of conduction in presynaptic terminals, at all levels of the central nervous system, represents one of the mechanisms of action of the barbiturate anaesthetic agents including methohexitone.

Summary

Methohexitone is a drug which has been investigated as thoroughly as any other intravenous drug for induction of anaesthesia. It provides advantages in terms of rapid recovery, minimal cardiovascular depression, and relatively few cumulative effects; it is less irritant to the tissues than other commonly used intravenous agents and is suitable for intramuscular use in children. A further advantage of methohexitone is its high potency. As an intravenous anaesthetic agent methohexitone provides a good balance between ease of anaesthetic control on the one hand, and rapid recovery on the other, and on the evidence presented would appear to be the best all purpose induction agent currently available.

Zusammenfassung

Methohexital ist ein Arzneimittel, das ebenso gründlich wie andere intravenöse Mittel zur Anaesthesie-Einleitung untersucht wurde. Es bietet Vorzüge hinsichtlich einer raschen Erholung, minimaler Herz-Kreislauf-Depression und relativ geringer kumulativer Effekte; es reizt die Gewebe weniger als andere häufig verwendete intravenöse Mittel und eignet sich auch zur intramuskulären Verabreichung bei Kindern. Ein weiterer Vorteil von Methohexital ist seine hohe Wirksamkeit. Als intravenöses Anaesthetikum gewährleistet es ein gutes Gleichgewicht zwischen leichter Anaesthesie-Kontrolle einerseits und rascher Erholung andererseits. Aufgrund der dargelegten Befunde scheint Methohexital das beste Allzweck-Einleitungsanaesthetikum zu sein, das heute zur Verfügung steht.

References

ANDERSEN, P., ECCLES, J. C., SEARS, T. A.: Cortically evoked depolarisation of primary afferent fibres of the spinal cord. J. Neurophysiol. 27, 63 (1964).

BARLOW, M. B., GOTTLICH, J.: The use of methohexital to shorten safely the hospitalisation of day cases. Med. Proc. 8, 458 (1962).

BARRON, D. W., DUNDEE, J. W.: The recently introduced rapidly acting barbiturates; a review and critical appraisal in relation to thiopentone. Brit. J. Anaesth. 33, 81 (1961).

BARRY, C. T., RENNIE, G. G., MACPHERSON, M. M.: Methohexitone sodium in anaesthesia for cystoscopy. Anaesthesia 17, 176 (1962).

BITTRICH, N. M., KANE, A. V. R., MOSHER, R. E.: Methohexital and its effect on liver function tests. Anaesthesiology 24, 81 (1963).

BRAND, L., MARK, L. C., SNELL, M. M., VRINDTEN, P., DAYTON, P. G.: Physiologic disposition of methohexital in man. Anaesthesiology 24, 331 (1963).

British Pharmacopoeia (B.P.) 1968, p. 603.

CHERNISH, S. M,. GRUBER, C. M., DeMEYER, M., LITTLEFIELD, S., STOELTING, V. K.: Double blind comparison of compound 22451, pentothal and surital. Fed. Proc. 15, 1333 (1956).

CLARKE, R. S. J., DUNDEE, J. W.: Clinical studies of induction agents XV. A comparison of the cumulative effects of thiopentone, methohexitone and propanidid. Brit. J. Anaesth. 38, 401 (1966).

— — BARRON, D. W., McARDLE, L.: Clinical studies of induction agents XXVI. The relative potencies of thiopentone, methohexitone and propanidid. Brit. J. Anaesth. 40, 593 (1968).

— — DAW, R. H.: Clinical studies of induction agents XI. The influence of some intravenous anaesthetics on the respiratory effects and sequelae of suxamethonium. Brit. J. Anaesth. 36, 307 (1964).

COHEN, S. M.: Accidential intra-arterial injection of drugs. Lancet 2, 361 (1948).

COLEMAN, D. J., DeVILLIERS, J. C.: Anaesthesia and Stereotactic surgery 19, 60 (1964).

COLEMAN, J., GREEN, R. A.: Methohexital, a short acting barbiturate. Anaesthesia 15, 411 (1960).

CONWAY, C. M., ELLIS, D. B., KING, N. W.: A comparison of the acute haemodynamic effects of thiopentone, methohexitone and propanidid in the dog. Brit. J. Anaesth. 40, 736 (1968).

CORSSEN, G., DOMINO, E. F.: Dissociative anaesthesia: Further pharmacologic studies and first clinical experience with the phencylidine derivative Cl-581. Anaesth. Analg. 45, 29 (1966).

DOBKIN, A. B., WYANT, G. M.: The physiological effect of intravenous anaesthesia on man. Canad. Anaesth. Soc. J. **4**, 295 (1957).

DOENICKE, A., KUGLER, J.: Electrical brain function during emergence time after methohexital and propanidid anaesthesia. Acta Anaesth. Scand. Suppl. 17, 99 (1965).

DRYDEN, G. E., MOSHIER, W.: Methohexital intramuscular for basal sedation. Appl. Ther. **5**, 521 (1963).

DUNDEE, J. W.: Comparison of the effects of methohexital and propanidid on the blood pressure. Acta Anaesth. Scand. Suppl. XVII, 51 (1965a).

— Comparison of side effects of methohexital and thiopental with propanidid. Acta Anaesth. Scand. Suppl. XVII, 77 (1965b).

— BARRON, D. W., KING, R.: The effect of methylation on the anaesthetic action of ethyl-methyl-propyl-thiobarbiturate. Brit. J. Anaesth. **32**, 566 (1960).

— CLARKE, R. S. J.: Clinical studies of induction agents XI: A comparative study of a new eugenol derivative F.B.A. 1420, with G29.505 and standard barbiturates. Brit. J. Anaesth. **36**, 100 (1964).

— MOORE, J.: Thiopentone and methohexital. A comparison as main anaesthetic agents for a standard operation. Anaesthesia **16**, 50 (1961a).

— — The effect of Scopolamine on methohexital anaesthesia. Anaesthesia **16**, 194 (1961b).

— RIDING, J. E.: A comparison of inactin and thiopentone as intravenous anaesthetics. Brit. J. Anaesth. **32**, 206 (1960).

— — BARRON, D. W., NICHOLL, R. M.: Some factors influencing the induction characteristics of methohexitone anaesthesia. Brit J. Anaesth. **33**, 296 (1961).

ECKENHOFF, J. E., HELRICH, M.: The effect of narcotics, thiopental and nitrous oxide upon respiration and respiratory responses to hypercapnia. Anaesthesiology **19**, 240 (1958).

EGBERT, L. D., OECH, S. R., ECKENHOFF, J. E.: Comparison of the recovery from methohexital and thiopental anaesthesia in man. Surg. Gynec. Obstet. **109**, 427 (1959).

ELLIOT, C. J. R., GREEN, R., HOWELLS, T. H., LONG, H. A.: Recovery from intravenous barbiturate anaesthesia: comparative study of recovery from methohexitone and thiopentone. Lancet **2**, 68 (1962).

FRANCIS, J. G.: Intra-arterial methohexitone. Anaesthesia **19**, 501 (1964).

GIBSON, W. R., DORAN, W. J., WOOD, W. C., SWANSON, E. E.: Pharmacology of stereoisomers of 1-methyl-5(1-methyl-2-pentynyl)-5-allyl-barbituric acid. J. Pharmacol. Exp. Ther. **125**, 23 (1959).

— SWANSON, E. E., DORAN, W. J.: Pharmacology of a short-acting non-sulphur barbituric acid derivative. Proc. Soc. exp. Biol. N.Y. **89**, 292 (1955).

GOLDMAN, V., HARRIS, P.: Intravenous induction of anaesthesia in the dental chair. Brit. Dent. J. **114**, 62 (1963).

GREEN, R. A.: Use of continuous methohexitone in general surgery. Symposium on methohexitone. May 1st and 2nd. Eli-Lilly & Co. 1969.

— JOLLY, C.: Methohexitone in dental anaesthesia. Brit. J. Anaesth. **32**, 593 (1960).

GRUBER, C. M., STOELTING, V. K., FORNEY, R. B., WHITE, P., DeMEYER, M.: Comparison of an ultrashort acting barbiturate (22451) with thiobarbiturates during anaesthesia. Anaesthesiology **18**, 50 (1957).

— — HICKS, M. L., DOUGHTY, S.: Clinical experiences during anaesthesia with a new short-acting barbiturate. Fed. Proc. **15**, 1407 (1956).

GUMPERT, J., PAUL, R.: Use of methohexitone for activation of the electro-encephalogram. Neurosurgical anaesthesists meeting, Sheffield 1970.

HANNINGTON-KIFF, J. G.: Measurement of recovery from outpatient general anaesthesia with a simple ocular test. Brit. Med. J. **3**, 132 (1970).

HEWITT, J. C., HAMILTON, R. C., O'DONNELL, J. F., DUNDEE, J. W.: Clinical studies of induction agents XIV: A comparative study of venous complications following thiopentone, methohexitone and propanidid. Brit. J. Anaesth. **38**, 115 (1966).

HOWELLS, T. H., HARNIK, E., KELLNER, G. A., ROSENOER, J. M.: Propanidid and methohexitone: Their comparative potency and narcotic action. Brit. J. Anaesth. **39**, 31 (1967).

JOHNSTONE, M., BARRON, P. T.: The cardiovascular effects of propanidid. A study in radiotelemetry. Anaesthesia **23**, 180 (1968).

JOLLY, C.: Recovery time from methohexitone anaesthesia. Brit. J. Anaesth. **32**, 576 (1960).

KIERSEY, D. K., BICKFORD, R. G., FAULCONER, A.: E.E.G. patterns produced by thiopental sodium during surgical operations: description and classification. Brit. J. Anaesth. **23**, 141 (1952).

KNAPP, M. R., BEECHER, H. K.: Post-anaesthetic nausea, vomiting and retching: evaluation of antiemetic drugs, dimenhydrinate (Dramamine), chlorpromazine and pentobarbital sodium. J. Amer. Med. Ass. **160**, 376 (1956).

LISCOMBE, R. M.: Methohexitone for tonsillectomy. A preliminary trial of intermittent methohexitone for tonsillectomy in children breathing air. Anaesthesia **23**, 268 (1968).

McMAHON, R. E.: The demethylation in vitro of N-methyl barbiturates and related compounds by mammalian liver microsomes. Biochem. Pharmacol. **12**, 1225 (1963).

MARSHALL, J. R.: Human antepartum passage of methohexital sodium. Obstet. and Gynec. **23**, 589 (1964).

MATHER, J. S., GOODHEAD, B.: Intra-arterial methohexitone and thiopentone. Anaesthesia **21**, 81 (1966).

MEAGHER, R. P.: Methohexital in conjunction with regional anaesthesia. Anaesth. Analg. **43**, 679 (1964).

MELZACK, R., WALL, P. D.: Pain mechanisms: a new theory. Science **150**, 971 (1965).

MENDELL, L. M., WALL, P. D.: Presynaptic hyperpolarisation a role for fine afferent fibres. J. Physiol. **172**, 274 (1964).

MILLER, J. R., STOELTING, V. K.: A preliminary communication on the sleep-producing effect of intramuscular methohexitone sodium in the paediatric patient. Brit. J. Anaesth. **35**, 48 (1963).

— — DANN, M. W.: A preliminary report on the use of intramuscular methohexital sodium for paediatric anaesthesia. Anaesth. Analg. **40**, 573 (1961).

MOORE, J., DUNDEE, J. W.: Promethazine. Its influence on the course of thiopentone and methohexital anaesthesia. Anaesthesia **16**, 61 (1961).

PITTS, F. N., DESMARAIS, G. M., STEWART, W., SCHADERG, K.: Induction of anaesthesia with methohexital and thiopental in electroconvulsive therapy. The effect on the electrocardiogram and clinical observations in 500 consecutive treatments with each agent. New Eng. J. Med. **273**, 353 (1965).

PRICE, H. L.: A dynamic concept of the distribution of thiopental in the human body. Anaesthesiology **21**, 40 (1960).

— KOVNAT, P. J., SAFER, J. N., CONNIER, E. H., PRICE, M. L.: Uptake of thiopental by body tissues and its relation to the duration of narcosis. Clin. Pharmacol, Therap. **1**, 16 (1960).

RADNAY, P.: Effects of propanidid and methohexital on physiological systems. Acta Anaesth. Scand. Suppl. XVII, 49 (1965).

REDISH, C. H., VORE, R. E., CHERNISH, S. M., GRUBER, C. M.: A comparison of thiopental sodium, methiural sodium and methohexital sodium in oral surgery patients. Oral Surg. **11**, 603 (1958).

RICHENS, A.: Microelectrode studies in the frog isolated spinal cord during depression by general anaesthetic agents. Brit. J. Pharmacol. **36**, 294 (1969a).

— The action of general anaesthetic agents on root responses of the frog isolated spinal cord. Brit. J. Pharmacol. **36**, 312 (1969b).

RIFFIN, I. M.: Methohexital sodium, a new induction anaesthetic, scientific exhibit. International Anaesthesiology research society meeting. Washington, D.C., April 4–7 (1960).

ROBSON, J. G., DAVENPORT, H. T., SUGIYAMA, R.: Differentiation of two types of pain by anaesthetics. Anaesthesiology **26**, 31 (1965).

ROWLANDS, D. E.: Comments on injection pain. Symposium on methohexitone. Eli Lilly & Co. May 1st and 2nd 1969.

RULE, D. C., WINTER, G. B., GOLDMAN, V., BROOKES, R. C.: Restorative treatment for children under general anaesthesia. The treatment of apprehensive and handicapped children as clinic outpatients. Brit. Dent. J. **123**, 480 (1967).

SANKAWA, H.: Cardiovascular effects of propanidid and methohexital sodium in dogs. Acta Anaesth. Scand. Suppl. XVII, 55 (1965).

STOELTING, V. K.: The use of a new intravenous oxygen barbiturate 25398 for intravenous anaesthesia (A preliminary report). Anaesth. Analg. **36**, 49 (1957).

SUNSHINE, I., WHITWAM, J. G., FIKE, W., FINKLE, B., LEBEAU, J.: Distribution and excretion of methohexitone in man. A study using gas and thin layer chromatography. Brit. J. Anaesth. **38**, 23 (1966).

SWERDLOW, M.: Dose duration effects of methohexitone. Symposium on methohexitone. Eli Lilly & Co. May 1st to 2nd 1969.

— MOORE, B. A.: A dose duration trial with propanidid. Brit. J. Anaesth. **39**, 573 (1967).

— — A dose duration study with methohexitone. Brit. J. Anaesth. **41**, 54 (1969).

TABERN, D. L., VOLWILER, E. H.: N-alkyl and N-aryl substituted barbituric acid. J. Amer. Chem. Soc. **58**, 1354 (1935).

TAYLOR, C., STOELTING, V. K.: Methohexital sodium. – A new ultrashort acting barbiturate. Anaesthesiology **21**, 29 (1960).

TEPFER, M., DRYDEN, G. E., CREGGER, I.: Methohexital sodium drip intravenously for head and neck surgery. J. Oral. Surg. **22**, 215 (1964).

United States National Formulary XII. p. 368.

WALL, P. D.: The laminar organisation of dorsal horn and effects of descending impulses. J. Physiol. **188**, 403 (1967).

WELLES, J. S., McMAHON, R. E., DORAN, W. J.: The metabolism and excretion of methohexital in the rat and dog. J. Pharmacol. Exp. Ther. **139**, 166 (1963).

WEYL, R., UNAL, B., ALPER, Y.: Clinical evaluation of a new ultra short acting oxygen barbiturate for intravenous anaesthesia. Surg. Gynec. Obstet. **107**, 588 (1958).

WHITWAM, J. G.: Lecture in Third Biennial conference on dental anaesthesia. Inst. Dental Surgery – Eastman Dental Hospital (1965).

— A clinical comparison of the incidence and duration of apnoea following methohexitone and thiopentone. Brit. J. Anaesth. **34**, 729 (1962).

— MANNERS, J. M.: Clinical comparison of thiopentone and methohexitone. Brit. Med. J. **1**, 1663 (1962).

WOODRUFF, R. A., PITTS, F. N., MacCLURE, J. N.: The drug modification of E.C.T. Arch. Gen. Psychiat. **18**, 605 (1968).

WYANT, G. M., CHANG, C. A.: Sodium methohexitone: a clinical study. Canad. Anaesth. Soc. J. **6**, 40 (1959).
— DOBKIN, A. B., AASHEIM, G. M.: Comparison of seven intravenous anaesthetic agents in man. Brit. J. Anaesth. **29**, 194 (1957).
YOUNG, D. S., WHITWAM, J. G.: Observations on dental anaesthesia introduced with methohexitone. I. Induction of Anaesthesia. Brit. J. Anaesth. **36**, 31 (1964a).
— — Observations on dental anaesthesia introduced with methohexitone. II Maintenance and recovery. Brit. J. Anaesth. **36**, 94 (1964b).
ZINDLER, M.: Changes of respiration and blood gases after propanidid. Acta Anaesth. Scand. Suppl. XVII, 7 (1965).

Myocardkontraktilität und Hämodynamik im Verlauf einer Methohexital-Narkose

Von **D. Soga** und **R. Beer**

Aus dem Institut für Anaesthesiologie der Universität München
(Vorstand: Prof. Dr. R. BEER)

Eine narkosebedingte Kreislaufdepression kann sowohl durch eine Beeinträchtigung der kardialen Pumpfunktion als auch durch eine Störung der peripheren Regulationsmechanismen hervorgerufen werden. Von besonderem Interesse ist natürlich die Kenntnis, in welchem Ausmaß eine Minderung der Myokardkontraktilität an einer Kreislaufdepression beteiligt ist. Die zur Beurteilung der Kreislaufwirkung eines Narkotikums bisher vielfach benutzte Messung des Herzminuten – bzw. Schlagvolumens sagt jedoch nur wenig über den kontraktilen Zustand des Herzens aus, da Änderungen der Inotropie durch gegensinnige hämodynamische Regulation, so z.B. durch Änderungen des venösen Rückflusses, kaschiert werden können. Erst im letzten Jahrzehnt gelang es, basierend auf den richtungsweisenden Arbeiten von SIEGEL und SONNENBLICK [3, 4], die Myokardkontraktilität auch am intakten Herzen genauer zu definieren und zahlenmäßig zu erfassen. Durch neue technische Errungenschaften ist es jetzt auch möglich Kontraktilitätsparameter am Menschen zu bestimmen.

Bezüglich ihrer Einwirkung auf die Myokardkontraktilität interessierten uns nun im besonderen Maße die zwei heute gebräuchlichsten ultrakurzwirkenden intravenösen Narkotika Methohexital (Brevimytal-Na = Brietal-Na der Firma Lilly) und Propanidid (Epontol der Firma Bayer). Bereits in vorausgegangenen Untersuchungen hatten wir nämlich den Einfluß dieser beiden Mittel auf die myokardiale Inotropie unter Verwendung des hierfür klassischen Verfahrens am isolierten Papillarmuskel getestet [5]. Diese Untersuchungen hatten ergeben, daß Methohexital und Propanidid in gleicher Konzentration eine fast gleich starke negativ inotrope Wirkung entfalten. Zur Beantwortung der Frage, welches Narkotikum nun tatsächlich bei der klinischen Anwendung eine stärkere Kontraktilitätsdepression hervorruft, muß jedoch folgendes berücksichtigt werden: Zur Erreichung des Toleranzstadiums wird bekanntlich eine weit geringere Dosis von Methohexital als von Propanidid benötigt. Ein Vergleich der Meßwerte von SUNSHINE u. Mitarb. [6] für Methohexital mit den Angaben von

DOENICKE u. Mitarb. [1] für Propanidid zeigt auch, daß während eines beträchtlichen Zeitabschnittes im Narkoseverlauf die Blutkonzentration von Methohexital deutlich unterhalb derjenigen von Propanidid liegt. In Anbetracht dieser Verhältnisse und aufgrund unserer Untersuchungsergebnisse am Papillarmuskel war es leicht vorstellbar, daß bei der klinischen Anwendung von Methohexital tatsächlich mit einer geringeren Beeinträchtigung der Myokardkontraktilität zu rechnen ist. Um nun zu klären, inwieweit diese Vermutung wirklich zutrifft, haben wir jetzt Untersuchungen am Herzen in situ durchgeführt.

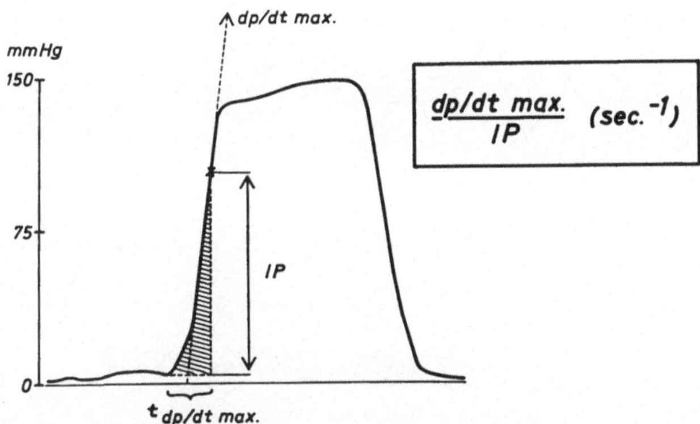

Abb. 1. Bestimmung des „Kontraktilitätsindex" dp/dt max./IP nach VERAGUT und KREYENBÜHL

In diesen Untersuchungen haben wir zur Erfassung der linksventrikulären Kontraktilität den „Kontraktilitätsindex" nach VERAGUT und KREYENBÜHL verwendet [2, 7]. Bei diesem Verfahren (Abb. 1) wird am linksventrikulären Druckablauf die maximale isolvolumetrische Druckanstiegsgeschwindigkeit (dp/dt max.) und der zu diesem Zeitpunkt erreichte augenblickliche Ventrikeldruck, instantaneous developed pressure, kurz IP genannt, bestimmt. Aus diesen beiden Größen wird dann der Quotient $\frac{dp/dt\ max.}{IP}$, der sogenannte „Kontraktilitätsindex" gebildet. Dieser Index ist von hämodynamischen Einflüssen vollkommen unabhängig [7]. Da sich andererseits mit ihm Änderungen der Inotropie gut und immer wieder reproduzierbar erfassen lassen, wird er heute als zweckmäßigster Parameter zur Beurteilung der Myokardkontraktilität am intakten Organismus angesehen. Voraussetzung für die Bestimmung des „Kontraktilitätsindex" ist jedoch, daß die linksventrikulären Druckkurven amplitudenmäßig und im zeitlichen Ablauf getreu aufgezeichnet werden. Dies ist aber nur mit Hilfe eines in der letzten Zeit entwickelten Spezialkatheters möglich (Abb. 2), bei welchem das Manometer an der Katheterspitze montiert ist (Abb. 3). Mit einem solchen Kathetertipmanometer erfolgt also die Druckaufnahme direkt intrakardial.

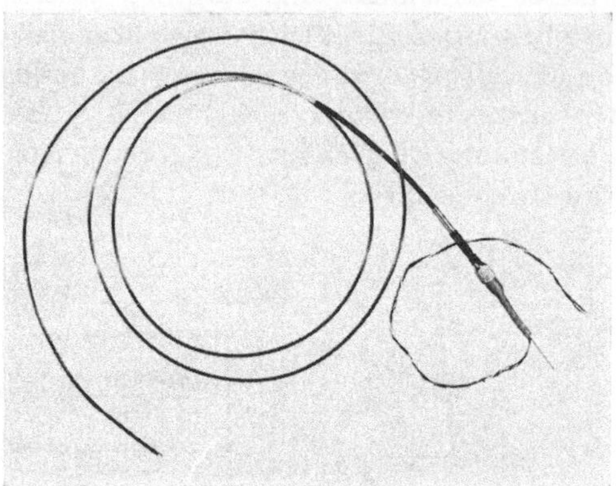

Abb. 2. Kathetertipmanometer MCP-055-5F der Firma Kulite

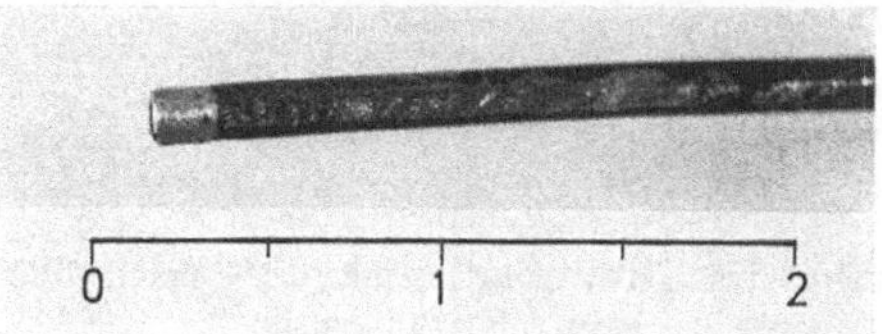

Abb. 3. Proximales Ende des Kathetertipmanometers

Um nun zu klären, wie das Methohexital und vergleichsweise Propanidid am intakten Herzen auf die Myokardkontraktilität und die wichtigsten hämodynamischen Parameter wirkt, haben wir zunächst unsere Untersuchungen am Hund durchgeführt. Die Versuchstiere befanden sich in Lachgasanalgesie und wurden kontrolliert beatmet. Nach Anlegen von EKG-Nadelelektroden wurden folgende Katheter placiert: 2 venöse Vorhof-Katheter zur Messung des zentralvenösen Druckes bzw. zur Farbstoffinjektion für die HZV-Bestimmung, 1 arterieller Katheter bis zur Aortenwurzel zur Aufnahme der Farbstoffverdünnungskurven und Messung des Aortendruckes und schließlich 1 Kathetertipmanometer in die linke Herzkammer zur Registrierung des linksventrikulären Druckablaufes. Mit dieser Versuchsanordnung konnten folgende Parameter gemessen bzw. berechnet werden: Herzminutenvolumen und Schlagindex, aortaler und zentralvenöser Blutdruck, Herzfrequenz, Gesamtgefäßwiderstand und schließlich der „Kontraktilitätsindex" $\dfrac{dp/dt\ max.}{IP}$. Nach Aufnahme der

Kontrollwerte wurden Methohexital bzw. Propanidid in einer Dosierung von 10 bzw. 40 mg/kg Körpergewicht in 30 sec verabreicht. Die angegebene Dosierung wird in der Veterinärmedizin üblicherweise zur Narkose beim Hund angewandt [8, 9].

Die für Methohexital erhobenen Befunde gibt die Abbildung 4 wieder. Der gleich zu Beginn auftretende Blutdruckabfall (Ao.$_m$) ist hier hauptsächlich durch eine erhebliche Minderung des Gesamtgefäßwiderstandes (R.ges.) bedingt. Die Abnahme der Myocardkontraktilität $\dfrac{dp/dt\ max.}{IP}$.

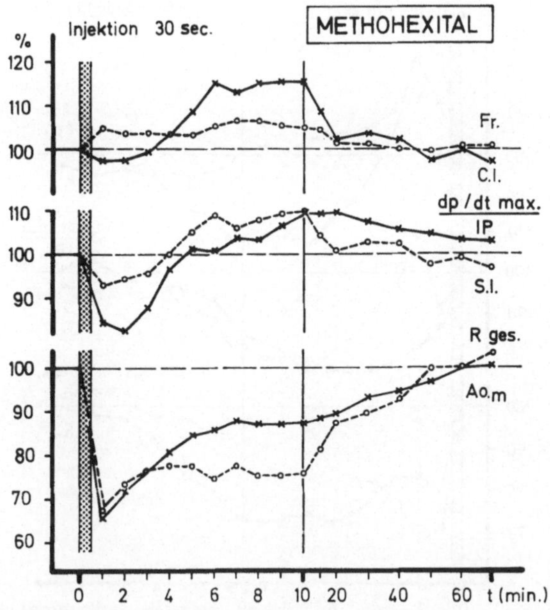

Abb. 4. Verhalten der Kreislaufparameter beim Hund nach Gabe von 10 mg/kg Körpergewicht Methohexital (n = 6)

ist dagegen verhältnismäßig gering ausgeprägt und vor allem von sehr kurzer Dauer. Zwischen der 4. und 5. min hat die Kontraktilität ihren Ausgangswert bereits wieder erreicht und übersteigt denselben in der anschließenden Periode. Das synchrone Verhalten des Schlag- (S.I.) und Herzindex (C.I.) trägt ab der 4. min dazu bei, daß der mittlere Aortendruck trotz der langanhaltenden Weitstellung der Gefäße wieder ansteigt.

Ganz anders verhalten sich die Kreislaufparameter in der Propanidid-Narkose (Abb. 5). Die stärkste Kreislaufdepression besteht hier zwischen der 5. und 7. min. Nach der initialen für Propanidid typischen Frequenz- und HZV-Steigerung beträgt der Cardiac Index in diesem Zeitabschnitt nur noch 78%, der Schlagindex 76% und der mittlere Aortendruck 72% des Ausgangswertes. Diese Depression ist, wie der Verlauf des „Kontraktilitätsindex" zeigt, im wesentlichen durch eine Abnahme der myokardialen Inotropie und kaum durch Änderung des Gefäßwiderstandes bedingt. Der Gefäßwiderstand fällt zwar initial als Antwort auf die stattgefundene Steigerung des Herzminutenvolumens deutlich ab, nähert sich aber zum Zeitpunkt der tiefsten Kreislaufdepression schon wieder dem Normbereich.

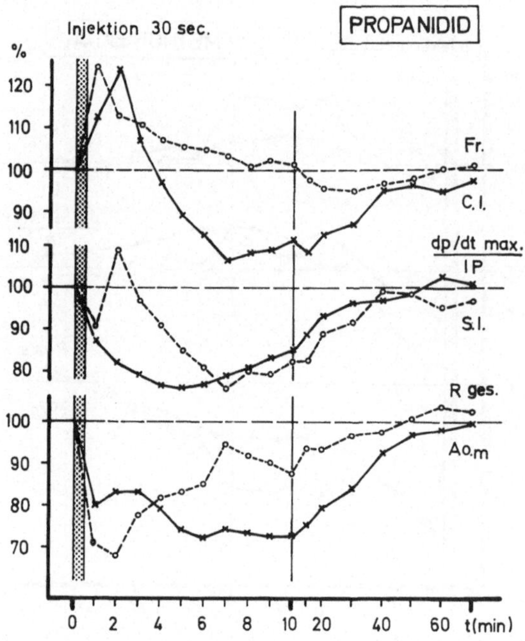

Abb. 5. Verhalten der Kreislaufparameter beim Hund nach Gabe von 40 mg/kg Körpergewicht Propanidid (n = 7)

Vergleicht man nun die Wirkung der beiden geprüften Narkotika auf die Myokardkontraktilität (Abb. 6), so ist es klar ersichtlich, daß bei der Verabreichung von klinischen Dosen das Herz durch Methohexital weniger beeinträchtigt wird als durch Propanidid, also unsere aufgrund der Papillarmuskelversuche aufgestellte Vermutung wirklich zutrifft.

Im letzten Teil unserer Arbeit untersuchten wir die Kreislaufwirkung von Methohexital und Propanidid während ihrer klinischen Anwendung am Menschen. Die Messungen fanden im Rahmen der üblichen Narkoseeinleitung statt. Bestimmt wurden die gleichen Kreislaufparameter wie in der vorangegangenen Untersuchungsreihe. Zur Aufnahme der linksventriku-lären Druckkurven wurde hier das Kathetertipmanometer (Abb. 7) über die rechte Arteria radialis eingebracht. Die beiden Narkotika wurden jeweils in klinisch üblicher Dosierung verabreicht, nämlich Methohexital 2 mg/kg bzw. Propanidid 7 mg/kg Körpergewicht.

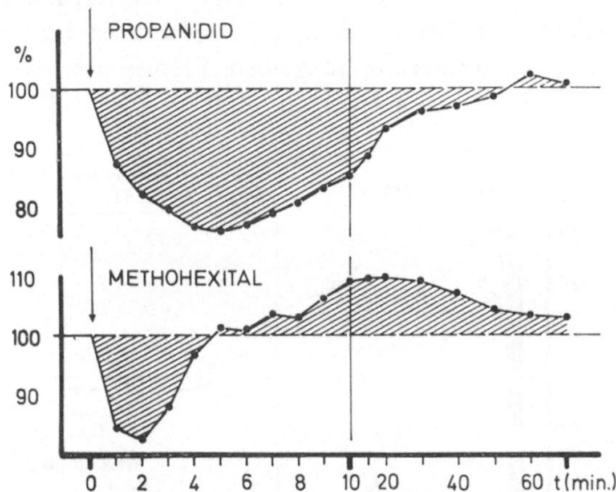

Abb. 6. Vergleich der Wirkung von Propanidid und Methohexital auf die Myokardkontraktilität beim Hund

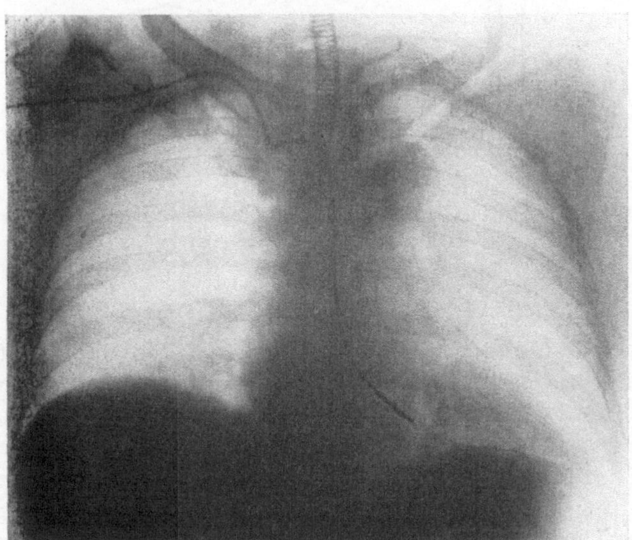

Abb. 7. Retrograd eingeführtes Kathetertipmanometer zur Aufnahme links-ventrikulärer Druckkurven beim Menschen in situ

Die Ergebnisse für Methohexital gibt die Abbildung 8 wieder. Wie man sieht, verhalten sich die Kreislaufparameter während der Methohexital-Narkose beim Menschen ähnlich wie beim Ganztier. Ganz im Vordergrund steht wiederum eine deutliche und langanhaltende Minderung des Gefäßwiderstandes. Daß der arterielle Mitteldruck trotzdem im Normbereich verbleibt, ist zunächst der geringfügigen und nur 2 min anhaltenden Kontraktilitätsdepression zu verdanken. Das Herz ist hier fähig, auf die durch Barorezeptorenstimulation ausgelöste Frequenzsteigerung mit einer Steigerung des Herzindex zu antworten.

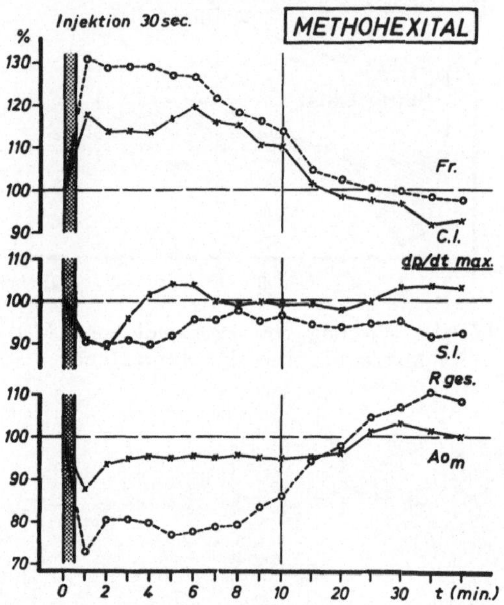

Abb. 8. Verhalten der Kreislaufparameter bei 6 Kranken nach Gabe von 2 mg/kg Körpergewicht Methohexital

Dagegen ist auch beim Menschen die Kreislaufdepression während der Propanidid-Narkose auf andere Ursachen zurückzuführen (Abb. 9). Der unmittelbar nach der Injektion stattfindende Abfall des arteriellen Mitteldruckes ist hier wiederum weniger durch Abnahme des Gefäßwiderstandes sondern vielmehr durch eine erhebliche Myokarddepression bedingt. Die für Propanidid typische initiale Frequenzsteigerung vermochte hier nicht wegen der starken Minderung der myokardialen Inotropie einen Abfall des Herzminutenvolumens zu verhindern. Bemerkenswert ist es, daß der „Kontraktilitätsindex" in der Erholungsphase nicht zum Ausgangswert zurückkehrt, sondern weiterhin vermindert bleibt.

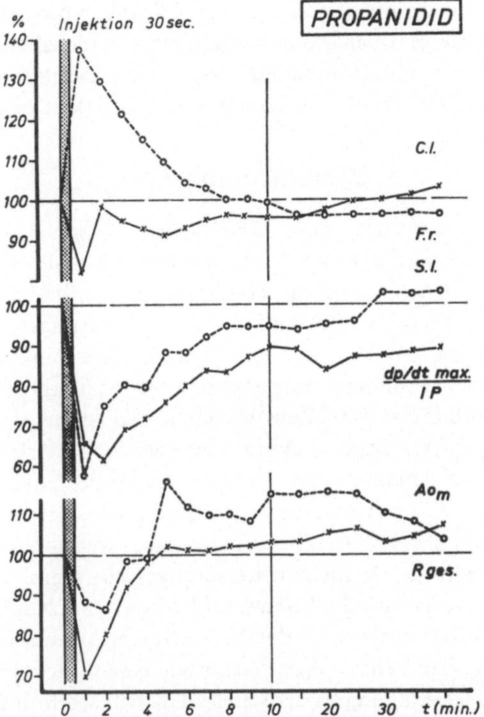

Abb. 9. Verhalten der Kreislaufparameter bei 6 Kranken nach Gabe von 7 mg/kg Körpergewicht Propanidid

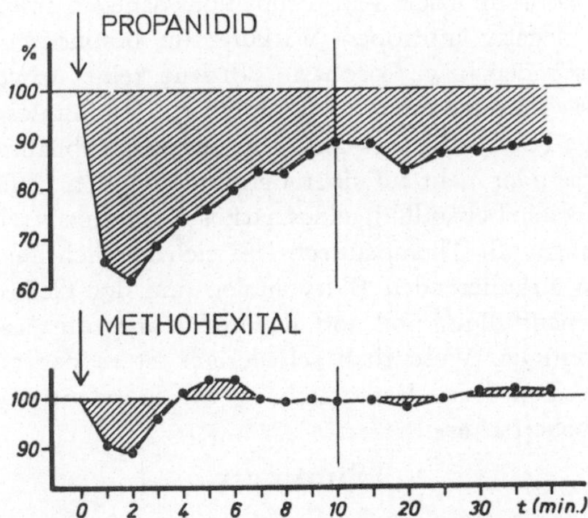

Abb. 10. Vergleich der Wirkung von Propanidid (7 mg/kg Körpergewicht) und Methohexital (2 mg/kg Körpergewicht) auf die Myokardkontraktilität beim Menschen

Eine direkte Gegenüberstellung des Effektes vom Methohexital und Propanidid auf die Myokardkontraktilität beim Menschen (Abb. 10) zeigt eindrucksvoll, wie unterschiedlich doch zwei Narkotika mit klinisch gleichem Indikationsbereich die Kontraktionsfähigkeit des Herzens beeinträchtigen können.

Zusammenfassung

Zusammenfassend führen unsere Untersuchungsergebnisse zu folgenden Feststellungen : Die aufgrund der Papillarmuskelversuche aufgestellte Hypothese, daß bei klinischer Anwendung die Myokardkontraktilität durch Methohexital weniger beeinträchtigt sein wird als durch Propanidid, hat sich sowohl in Untersuchungen am Ganztier als auch in Messungen am Menschen bestätigt. In beiden Untersuchungsgruppen führte Methohexital im Gegensatz zu Propanidid nur zu einer mäßigen Abnahme der myokardialen Inotropie. Die durch Methohexital verursachte Kreislaufdepression ist vor allem auf eine Abnahme des Gefäßwiderstandes zurückzuführen. Die am Ganztier für Methohexital und Propanidid gewonnenen Ergebnisse sind grundsätzlich gut auf den Menschen übertragbar, wenngleich auch die durch Methohexital bedingte Kontraktilitätsdepression beim Menschen noch geringer und diejenige durch Propanidid bedingte noch stärker ausgeprägt war als am Ganztier. Aufgrund der beobachteten unterschiedlichen Herzkreislaufwirkung der beiden Kurznarkotika lassen sich für die klinische Praxis folgende Überlegungen anstellen: Da bei Methohexital eine Weitstellung der Gefäße im Vordergrund steht, sollte man dieses Mittel bei Kranken mit bestehendem Volumenmangel nur mit Vorsicht, am besten erst nach Volumenauffüllung anwenden. Bei Kranken im Schock dürfte Methohexital kontraindiziert sein. Propanidid dagegen sollte wegen seiner ausgeprägten negativ inotropen Wirkung im besonderen bei Kranken mit Myokardschäden bzw. Coronarinsuffizienz keine Anwendung finden. Letztlich ist das Wissen darum, ob die durch ein bestimmtes Narkosemittel hervorgerufene Kreislaufdepression mehr auf einer Abnahme der myokardialen Inotropie oder mehr auf einer Verminderung des Gefäßwiderstandes beruht, auch für die Behandlung eines narkosebedingten Kreislaufzwischenfalles bedeutungsvoll. Therapeutisch läßt sich nämlich ein Mißverhältnis zwischen dem zirkulierenden Blutvolumen und der Gefäßweitenstellung durch Volumenauffüllung und notfalls durch Gabe von Vasokonstriktoren recht gut beseitigen. Wesentlich schwieriger ist es dagegen, eine akute Myokarddepression durch Verabreichung von inotropiesteigernden Medikamenten zu beherrschen.

Summary

Basing on the results obtained in experiments using the papillary muscle, the hypothesis was put forward that, in clinical application, methohexital would probably impair myocardial contractility to a lesser extent than would propanidide. We have confirmed this assumption both in studies on the intact animal and in measurements in the human being. Unlike propanidide, methohexital produced no more than a moderate reduction of myocardial inotropism in either experimental group. The circulatory depression induced by methohexital is mainly due to a reduction of the vascular resistance. On principle, the results gained with methohexital and with propanidide in the intact animal are well applicable to the human, although the depression of contractility induced by methohexital was even less pronounced in the human, while that evoked by propanidide in the human was more distinct than in the intact animal. In view of the differences observed in the cardiac and circulatory effects of these two shortacting anaesthetics, the following theories may be deduced with regard to clinical practice: since in methohexital the vasodilator effect is predominant, this drug should be given only with caution to patients with deficient blood volume, and preferably only after having filled up the volume. In patients with shock it will probably be contraindicated. By contrast, propanidide should not be applied to patients with myocardial damage or coronary failure because of its pronounced negative inotropic effect. For adequate treatment of anaesthesia-induced incidents it is important to know whether the circulatory depression caused by a certain anaesthetic is due rather to a decrease in the myocardial inotropism or more probably to a reduction of the vascular resistance, since disproportions arising between the volume of the circulating blood and the degree of vasodilation are readily reversed by filling up the volume and, if necessary, by administration of vasoconstrictor drugs. On the other hand, it is considerably more difficult to control acute myocardial depression by administration of inotropism-increasing drugs.

Literatur

1. DOENICKE, A., KRUMEY, I., KUGLER, J., KLEMPA, J.: Experimental Studies of the Breakdown of Epontol: Determination of Propanidid in human Serum. Brit. J. Anaesth. **40**, 415 (1968).
2. KREYENBÜHL, H. P.: Die Dynamik und Kontraktilität des linken Ventrikels. Basel (Schweiz)-New York: S. Karger-Verlag 1969.
3. SIEGEL, J. H., SONNENBLICK, E. H.: Isometric Time-Tension Relationships as an Index of Myocardial Contractility. Circ. Res. **12**, 597 (1963).
4. — — The Quantification of Myocardial Contractility in Dog and Man. Cardiologia **45**, 189 (1964).
5. SOGA, D., BRECHTELSBAUER, H., BEER, R.: Wirkung von Propanidid, Methohexital und Halothane auf die isometrische Kontraktion des isolierten Herzmuskels. Z. prakt. Anästh. (im Druck).
6. SUNSHINE, I., WHITWAM, J. G., FIKE, W. W., FINKLE, B., LeBEAU, J.: Distribution and Excretion of Methohexitone in Man. Brit. J. Anaesth. **38**, 33 (1966).

7. Veragut, O. P., Kreyenbühl, H. P.: Estimation and Quantification of Myocardial Contractility in the Closed-chest Dog. Cardiologia **47**, 96 (1965).
8. Welles, J. S., McMahon, R. E., Doran, W. J.: The Metabolism and Excretion of Methohexital in the Rat and Dog. J. Pharm. Exo. Therap. **2**, 166 (1963).
9. Wirth, W., Hoffmeister, F.: Pharmakologische Untersuchungen mit Propanidid. Anaesthesiologie und Wiederbelebung **4**, 17. Berlin-Heidelberg-New York: Springer 1965.

Vergleichende mechanokardiographische Untersuchungen intravenöser Kurznarkotica

Von **A. Hartung**

Aus der Anaesthesieabteilung (Chefarzt: Dr. CH. LEHMANN)
der Chirurg. Klinik und Poliklinik (Direktor: Prof. Dr. G. MAURER)
am Klinikum rechts der Isar der Technischen Universität München

Die Frage, ob und wieweit Kurznarkotika vom Typ der Barbiturate in üblicher Dosierung die Herzkraft vermindern, ist für die Narkose bei Patienten mit eingeschränkter kardialer Leistungsfähigkeit von besonderer Bedeutung.

ÅSTRÖM u. Mitarb. wiesen am isolierten Meerschweinchenherzen einen dosisabhängigen, negativ inotropen Effekt von Methohexital nach [1]. PICHLMAYR sah nach Thiopental in hoher Dosierung eine beträchtliche Abnahme des Herz-Zeit-Volumens [4]. Untersuchungen von DROST u. Mitarb. ergaben mit der gleichen Methode nach Methohexital keine eindeutigen Veränderungen [2]. Die Ergebnisse der Bestimmung von dp/dt von Frau SOGA haben Sie eben gehört.

Die unterschiedlichen Untersuchungsbedingungen, Dosierungen und Meßmethoden in den einzelnen Versuchsreihen erlauben bisher keine eindeutige Beantwortung der hier aufgeworfenen Fragen. Wir entschlossen uns deshalb zu einer vergleichenden Untersuchung von zwei der derzeit am häufigsten verwendeten Barbiturate, Methohexital und Thiopental.

Da wir uns beim Menschen, besonders im Rahmen einer experimentellen Narkose nicht zu direkten intraventriculären Druckmessungen entschließen konnten, wählten wir indirekte, mechanokardiographische Methoden. Die Prüfung der beiden Substanzen an der gleichen Gruppe herzgesunder Versuchspersonen erfolgte bei klar definierten und reproduzierbaren Ausgangsbedingungen und gleichbleibender kardialer Leistungsfähigkeit. Vagale Effekte wurden durch eine vorhergehende intravenöse Atropingabe von 0,5 mg ausgeschaltet. Diese Gegebenheiten ermöglichten echte statistische Analysen der Kreislaufeffekte im gepaarten Vergleich.

Die Versuche wurden an 3 Frauen und 12 Männern im Alter von 21 bis zu 28 Jahren unter Grundumsatzbedingungen in einem zeitlichen Abstand von mindestens einer Woche durchgeführt. Nach einer Ruheperiode von 20 min legten wir die Meßfühler zur Aufnahme des Carotispulses und der Atembewegungen, das Mikrophon für das Phonokardiogramm und die Elektroden zur Registrierung der Ableitung II des EKG's. an. Der zentrale Venendruck wurde nach röntgenologischer Kontrolle der Katheterlage durch einen von der V. basilica aus eingeführten Bard-Katheter über einen Statham-Meßwandler registriert, der Blutdruck auskultatorisch nach Riva-Rocci gemessen.

Nach Aufzeichnung der Kontrollwerte auf einem Schwarzer-6-fach-Schreiber erhielten die Patienten äquipotente Dosen, d. h. 1,5 mg/kg

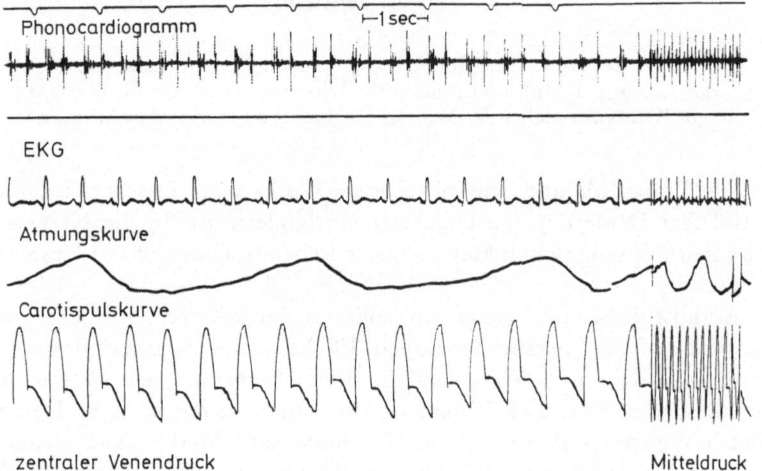

Abb. 1. Synchrone Aufzeichnung der mittelfrequenten Ableitung des Phonokardiogramms, der Ableitung II des Elektrokardiogramms, der Atmung, des Carotispulses und des zentralen Venendruckes bei einer Papiergeschwindigkeit von 25 mm/sec

Körpergewicht Methohexital oder 3,75 mg/kg Körpergewicht Thiopental. Um eine vergleichbare Verteilung bzw. Pharmakokinetik zu erzielen, wurde auf Einhaltung gleicher Injektionsgeschwindigkeiten geachtet.

Nach Gabe der beiden Testsubstanzen registrierten wir die einzelnen Meßgrößen unter Spontanatmung kontinuierlich über 5 min.

Die Abbildungen 1 und 2 zeigen eine synchrone Aufzeichnung der mittelfrequenten Ableitung des Phonokardiogramms, der Ableitung II des Elektrokardiogramms, der Atmung, des Carotispulses und des zentralen Venendruckes bei einer Papiergeschwindigkeit von 25 mm/sec und 50 mm/sec.

Wir bestimmten hieraus das Zeitintervall zwischen dem Beginn der elektrischen Kammererregung, d. h. dem Beginn der Q- bzw. R-Zacke im EKG und dem Beginn des Steilanstiegs im Carotispuls, das wir im folgenden als QA bezeichnen. Außerdem wurde der zeitliche Abstand zwischen Q und der ersten klar erkennbaren Schwingungsgruppe des 1. Herztones gemessen und als Q1 bezeichnet. Für jede dieser Meßgrößen werteten wir mindestens 4 Herzaktionen aus. Für die statistischen Berechnungen wurde das arithmetische Mittel verwendet.

Aus der Weg-Zeit-Kurve des Carotispulses bestimmten wir den Punkt der maximalen Aufstrichgeschwindigkeit. Er entspricht dem Gipfelpunkt der Kurve der 1. Differentialableitung dc/dt, die, wie Untersuchungen von SIMONYI und BANSAGHI zeigten, in enger Beziehung zu der Auswurfgeschwindigkeit des Blutes aus dem linken Ventrikel steht [5].

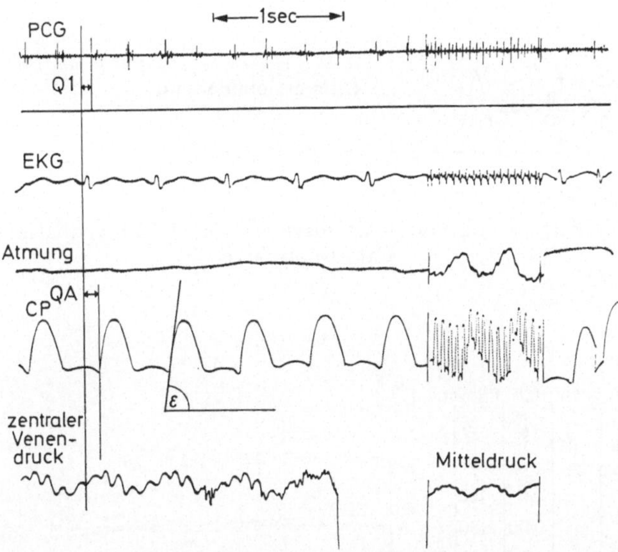

Abb. 2. Synchrone Aufzeichnung der mittelfrequenten Ableitung des Phonokardiogramms, der Ableitung II des Elektrokardiogramms, der Atmung, des Carotispulses und des zentralen Venendruckes bei einer Papiergeschwindigkeit von 50 mm/sec

Für die graphische Auswertung der folgenden Abbildungen verwendeten wir den Tangens des Steigungswinkels ε der Weg-Zeit-Kurve des Carotispulses. Das Zeitintervall zwischen dem Beginn der elektrischen Kammererregung und der Ankunft der Pulskurve in der Carotis bei gegebenem diastolischem Druck und bei konstanter Pulswellenlaufgeschwindigkeit ist nach LYDTIN u. Mitarb. ein indirektes Maß für die Druckanstiegsgeschwindigkeit [3].

Abbildung 4 faßt unsere Ergebnisse zusammen. Von oben nach unten sehen Sie systolischen Blutdruck, Herzfrequenz, QA-Zeit, Q1-Zeit und tg ε. Der systolische Blutdruck fällt nach Thiopental und Methohexital

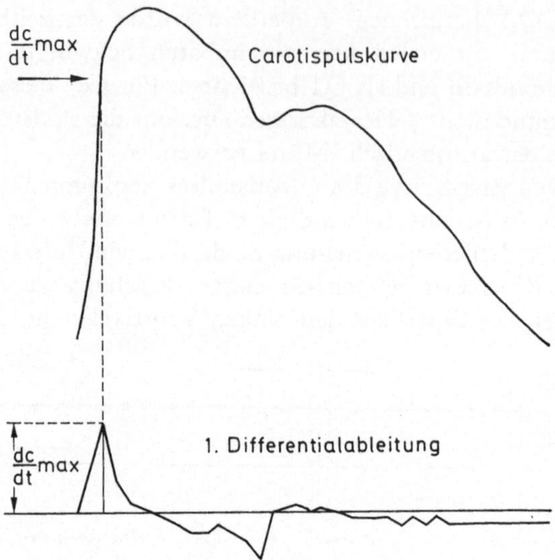

Abb. 3. Die Bestimmung von dc/dt max. aus der 1. Differentialableitung der Carotispulskurve

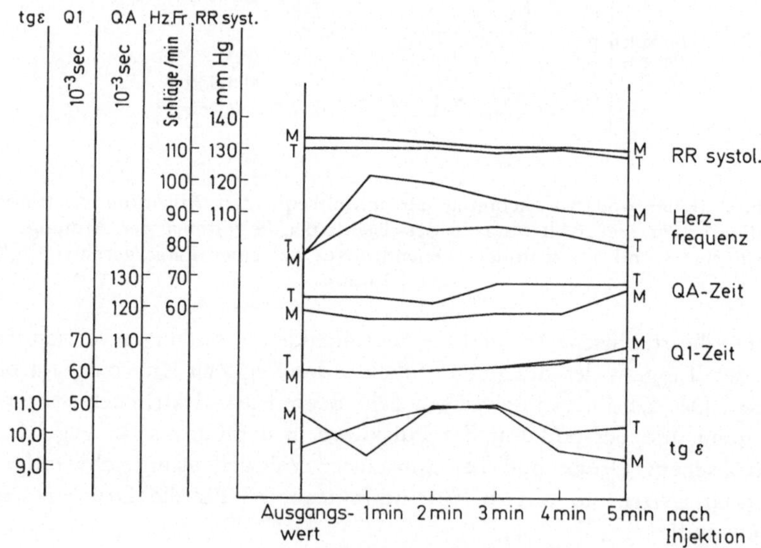

Abb. 4. Die Veränderungen von systolischem Blutdruck, Herzfrequenz, QA-Zeit, Q1-Zeit und tg ε nach Methohexital und Thiopental in minütlichen Messungen über 5 min

geringgradig ab. Auffallend ist vor allem der im Vergleich zu Thiopental stärkere Anstieg der Herzfrequenz nach Methohexitalgabe. QA-Zeit und Q1-Zeit zeigen richtungs- und auch größenordnungsmäßig ein weitgehend übereinstimmendes Verhalten. Der Tangens des Steigungswinkels der Carotispulskurve fällt nach Methohexital zunächst ab, um sich im weiteren Verlauf wieder mit den Werten für Thiopental zu treffen.

Wir sind uns bewußt, daß unsere Ergebnisse nur indirekte Indizien für die Beurteilung der kardialen Kontraktilität liefern. Andererseits weist die richtungsmäßige Übereinstimmung voneinander unabhängiger Meßgrößen, wie z. B. die Zunahme von QA bei gleichzeitiger Abnahme des Steigungswinkels des Carotispulses eindeutig darauf hin, daß der linke Ventrikel sich nach Gabe von Methohexital langsamer entleert. Von besonderer Bedeutung erscheint uns der Abfall von tg e in der 1. min nach Gabe von Methohexital bei gleichzeitigem Anstieg der Herzfrequenz.

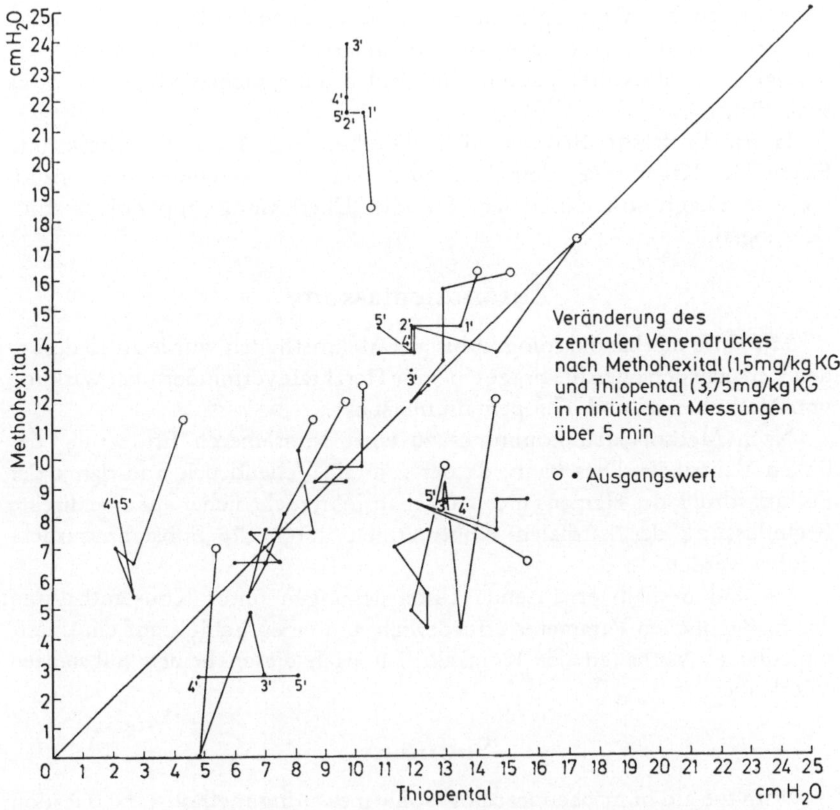

Abb. 5. Die Veränderung des zentralen Venendruckes nach Methohexital und Thiopental in minütlichen Messungen über 5 min

Abbildung 5 zeigt das Verhalten des zentralen Venendruckes. Die Abszisse gibt die Werte bei Thiopental, die Ordinate bei Methohexital wieder. Ohne Berücksichtigung der Details läßt sich hieraus eine eindeutige Tendenz zur Abnahme des Venendruckes nach beiden Substanzen ablesen.

Da unter Methohexital somit auch der Füllungsdruck des Herzens stärker absinkt, läßt sich aus der Abnahme von tg ε und der Zunahme von QA nicht direkt auf eine Beeinflussung der kardialen Kontraktilität durch das Pharmakon schließen. Es erscheint vielmehr wahrscheinlich, daß die Abnahme der Kontraktionsgeschwindigkeit entsprechend dem Starling-Mechanismus teilweise durch eine Abnahme des Füllungsdruckes mit konsekutiver Faserverkürzung zu erklären ist.

Aus diesem Grunde sind ergänzende Untersuchungen, bei denen das zentrale Blutangebot und evtl. auch die Herzfrequenz konstant gehalten werden, notwendig, bevor wir aus unseren Untersuchungen auf ein unterschiedliches Verhalten der Kontraktilität nach beiden Substanzen schließen dürfen.

Bei kritischer Wertung können wir aus unseren bis jetzt vorliegenden Ergebnissen noch nicht sicher auf eine unterschiedliche Beeinflussung der kardialen Kontraktilität durch die beiden untersuchten Kurznarkotika schließen.

Herrn Professor Blömer, dem Direktor der 1. Med. Klinik und Herrn Dr. Kiefhaber, dem Leitenden Arzt der Abteilung für Cardiologische Diagnostik danke ich für die Überlassung apparativer Einrichtungen.

Zusammenfassung

Mit Hilfe mechanokardiographischer Meßmethoden wurde an 15 gesunden Versuchspersonen die Frage einer die Herzkraft vermindernden Wirkung von Methohexital und Thiopental untersucht.

Nach Methohexital kommt es zu einer langsameren Entleerung des linken Ventrikels. Dies kann, da der zentrale Venendruck und damit der Füllungsdruck des Herzens hier stärker absinkt, nicht sicher auf eine direkte Beeinflussung der kardialen Kontraktilität durch die Substanz zurückgeführt werden.

Es sind deshalb ergänzende Untersuchungen unter Konstanthaltung der maßgeblichen Parameter erforderlich, um einen Schluß auf ein unterschiedliches Verhalten der Kontraktilität nach diesen beiden Substanzen zu erlauben.

Summary

With the aid of mechanocardiographic measuring methods, the question whether methohexital and thiopental exert reducing effects on the cardiac strength was examined on 15 healthy trial subjects.

Methohexital leads to a delay in the emptying of the left ventricle. Since there develops a pronounced drop in the central venous pressure and, accordingly, in the filling pressure of the heart this effect cannot conclusively be attributed to a direct influence of the substance on cardiac contractility.

Supplementary examinations with the relevant parameters kept constant will therefore be necessary, in order to elucidate whether these two substances produce different responses with regard to cardiac contractility.

Literatur

1. Åström, A., Bernhoff, A., Persson, N.-A.: Effects of Propanidid and Methohexital on the contractile force of the isolated Guinea-Pig Heart. Acta anaesth. Scand. **14**, 45–54 (1970).
2. Drost, R., Pichlmayr, I., Soga, D., Manz, R., Beer, R.: Vergleichende Untersuchungen über die Wirkung der Kurznarkotika Propanidid und Methohexital-Na auf das mittels Radiokardiographie gemessene Herzminutenvolumen. Anaesthesist **19**, 383 (1970).
3. Lydtin, H., Schnelle, K., Lohmöller, G., Zöllner, N.: Synchronous Recordings of Bcg, ECG, Carotid Pulse Wave, and PCG in Acute Pharmacological Trials. Ballistocardiography and Cardiovascular Therapy. Proc. 2nd World Congr. Ballistocard. cardiovasc. Dynamics, Oporto 1969; Bibl. cardiol. **26**, 36–41. Basel/München/New York: Karger 1970.
4. Pichlmayr, I.: Über den Einfluß verschiedener Narkosearten auf Durchblutung und Funktion der Leber sowie Durchblutung der Hirnrinde. Habil.-Schrift, München 1967.
5. Simonyi, J., Bansaghy, L.: Nyomas-éspulzusgörbek agyszerü elektronikus derivälasa. Orvos es Technika **4**, 119 (1966).

Puls-, Blutdruck- und EKG-Veränderungen bei Methohexital-Narkosen

Von **I. Wilckens** und **R. Roggenkämper**

Aus der Anaesthesie-Abteilung (Chefarzt: Dr. CH. LEHMANN)
der Chirurg. Klinik und Poliklinik (Direktor: Prof. Dr G. MAURER)
am Klinikum rechts der Isar der Technischen Universität München

Methohexital verdankt seine Anerkennung nicht zuletzt der Tatsache, daß es das Herz- und Kreislaufsystem kaum beeinträchtigt.

In der Literatur wurden bisher keine EKG-Veränderungen während einer Betäubung mit Methohexital beschrieben. Auch Blutdruckschwankungen, bei denen genauso häufig über leichte Anstiege wie über geringfügige Abfälle des systolischen Druckes berichtet wird, werden selten angegeben. Auffallend dagegen ist die von allen Autoren beobachtete deutliche Frequenzzunahme des Pulses. Man nimmt an, daß sie durch die dem Methohexital zugeschriebene parasympathikolytische Wirkung zustandekommt. Um dieser vagolytischen Komponente willen wird immer wieder diskutiert, ob man bei ambulanten Kurznarkosen unter Umständen auf eine Prämedikation verzichten dürfe.

Wir versuchten, die Auswirkungen des Methohexitals auf das Herz- und Kreislaufsystem mit Hilfe von Blutdruck-, Puls- und EKG-Messungen zu registrieren.

Methodik

Der Effekt des Methohexitals auf Blutdruck, Puls und EKG wurde in zwei getrennten Versuchsreihen gemessen.

Während der ersten beobachteten wir 30 gesunde Studenten und Studentinnen im Alter von 20–30 Jahren, während der zweiten 15 vorwiegend gesunde Patienten, entweder junge Frauen vor kleineren gynäkologischen Eingriffen oder ältere Kranke der urologischen Abteilung.

Bei allen Versuchen wurde auf eine Prämedikation verzichtet, um eine durch sie bedingte Wirkung auf Blutdruck und Puls auszuschließen.

Die Studenten erhielten 2 mg Methohexital pro kg Körpergewicht in einer 1%igen Lösung. 100 mg gaben wir als Initialdosis, den Rest verabreichten wir fraktioniert im Abstand von 3–4 min. Den Patienten injizierten wir die doppelte Menge, also 4 mg pro kg Körpergewicht. Zur

Einleitung der Narkose erhielten sie ebenfalls 100 mg und als Repetitionsdosen 20–40 mg bis zur errechneten Gesamtmenge.

Während der Messungen wurde von chirurgischen Handlungen abgesehen, um eine Auswirkung des Operationsstresses auf Blutdruck und Puls zu vermeiden.

Bei allen Versuchspersonen registrierten wir Blutdruck, Puls und EKG vor Beginn der Betäubung, unmittelbar nach der Injektion und in fortlaufenden Abständen von 2 min. Die Messungen wurden so lange fortgesetzt, bis die Studenten erwachten bzw. die Patienten ihre letzte Dosis erhalten hatten.

Die durchschnittliche Betäubungsdauer betrug bei den Studenten 4–10 min. Bei den Patienten wurde sie wegen der nachfolgenden Narkose zur Operation nicht bestimmt.

In den Fällen, in denen es nach der Injektion der Initialdosis oder im Laufe der Betäubung zur Apnoe kam, wurden die Versuchspersonen bis zum Wiedereinsetzen der Spontanatmung mit Sauerstoff ventiliert.

Ergebnisse

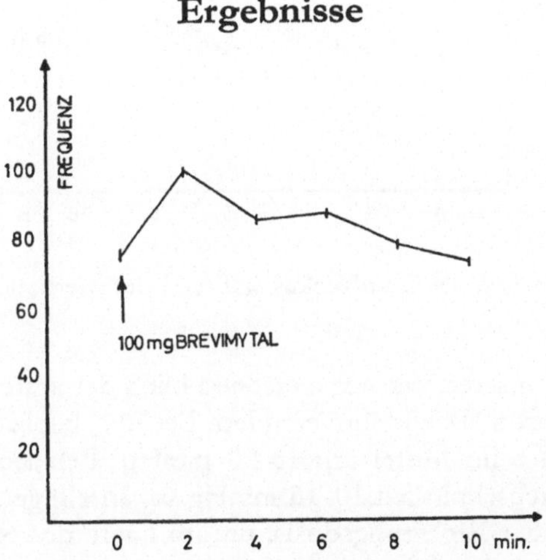

Abb. 1. Verhalten des Pulses während der Methohexital-Narkose

Bei der Betrachtung der Pulsveränderungen während der GesamtNarkosedauer fiel in beiden Versuchsreihen eine deutliche Pulsfrequenz-Steigerung auf. Meist erfolgte die stärkste Beschleunigung in den ersten 2 min. Seltener war ein verzögertes Ansteigen während der 4. bis 5. min. Der mittlere Frequenzanstieg betrug bei den Studenten 28,8 und bei den Patienten 25,7 Schläge pro min. Bei den letzteren wieder zeigten die älteren eine wesentlich geringere Zunahme als die jüngeren Kranken.

Die weiteren Ergebnisse lassen erkennen, daß bei den Studenten die Frequenz nach Erreichen ihres Höchstwertes kontinuierlich abfiel und beim Erwachen in den meisten Fällen ihren Ausgangswert erreichte oder sogar darunter sank.

Bei den Patienten fiel die Frequenz nach Erreichen des Höchstwertes ebenfalls ab, blieb aber fast immer höher als bei der Ausgangsmessung. Wahrscheinlich ist dieses Ergebnis durch die größere Gesamtdosis und die häufigen, fraktionierten Gaben von Methohexital zu erklären. Die Repetitionsdosis löst fast immer eine deutliche Erhöhung der Pulsfrequenz aus.

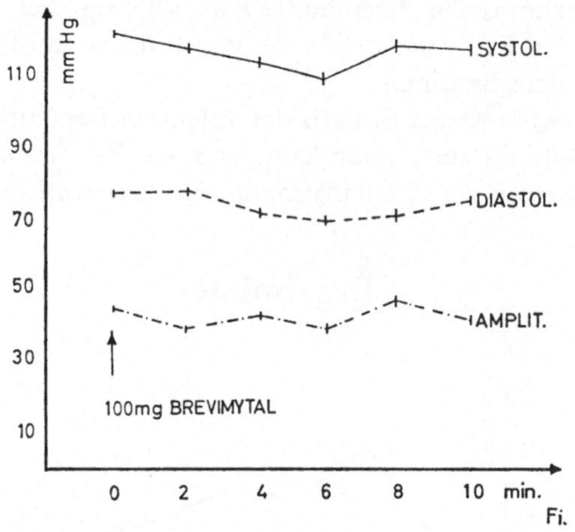

Abb. 2. Verhalten des Blutdruckes während der Methohexital-Narkose

Bei nur 5% unserer Versuchspersonen blieb der systolische Blutdruck während der ganzen Narkose unverändert. Bei 70% beobachteten wir einen Abfall des Wertes im Mittel um 10–20 mmHg. Bei den restlichen 25% nahm er um durchschnittlich 10–15 mmHg zu. In einigen Fällen stieg der Blutdruck nach der Einleitungsdosis, um im Laufe der Narkose bis unter den Ausgangswert abzufallen.

Weder der Abfall noch der Anstieg des systolischen Blutdruckes folgten der Initialdosis von Methohexital so unverzüglich wie die Pulsveränderungen. Meist wurden sie erst in einem zeitlichen Abstand von 4–5 min deutlich. Gegen Ende der Narkose näherte sich der systolische Wert der Ausgangslage. Häufig allerdings beharrte er nach Abfall auf einem etwas niedrigeren und nach Anstieg auf einem höheren Niveau.

Der diastolische Blutdruck war während der Narkose weniger starken Schwankungen unterworfen. In annähernd der gleichen Anzahl der Fälle kam es sowohl zu einem Anstieg als auch zu einem Abfall des Wertes.

Die Amplitude der diastolischen Schwankungen lag bei 5–10 mmHg. Die systolischen und diastolischen Veränderungen verliefen nicht unbedingt parallel. Es kann bei Anstieg und Abfall des systolischen Druckes ebensogut zu einer Zu- als auch zu einer Abnahme des diastolischen Wertes kommen.

Wenn wir die systolisch-diastolische Blutdruckamplitude berechnen, finden wir bei nur 16% aller Versuchspersonen ein unverändertes Verhältnis beider Größen. Bei 84%, also der überwiegenden Mehrzahl, nahm die Amplitude ab. Die Verminderung reichte von 5–40 und betrug durchschnittlich 10–15 mmHg. Meistens war sie durch die Senkung des systolischen, seltener durch einen Anstieg des diastolischen Blutdruckes bedingt. Aus diesem Grunde lief die Amplitudenabnahme der systolischen Senkung zeitlich parallel. Auch die Amplitudengröße erreichte bis zur Beendigung der Narkose annähernd ihren Ausgangswert.

Wir registrierten das EKG gleichzeitig mit Blutdruck und Puls und schrieben bei allen Versuchspersonen die zweite Standardableitung mit einer Geschwindigkeit von 50/sec.

Wie die Autoren vor uns, konnten auch wir während der Betäubung mit Methohexital keine EKG-Veränderungen beobachten. Es ist hier lediglich die schon bei den Pulsabweichungen besprochene Frequenzzunahme zu erwähnen. Wir sahen in keinem Fall eine Rhythmusstörung. Nur bei einem 70jährigen Patienten der urologischen Abteilung traten gegen Ende der Narkose 2 Extrasystolen auf. Auch nach Ansicht der Kardiologen ist ihr Entstehen nicht auf das Methohexital zurückzuführen.

Wir beobachteten keine Veränderungen der Vorhofserregung oder Verlängerung der Überleitungszeit. Der Kammerkomplex blieb in allen Fällen in Form und Dauer erhalten. Es trat bei keiner der Versuchspersonen eine Störung der Erregungsrückbildung auf.

Diskussion

Versucht man die in unseren Meßreihen erhaltenen Ergebnisse mit den bereits aus der Literatur bekannten Wirkungen des Methohexitals zu erklären, gelingt dies am einfachsten bei der Auswertung der Pulsveränderungen. Wie wir schon in der Einleitung erwähnten, wird dem Methohexital eine vagolytische Komponente zugeschrieben, die als Ursache für den Frequenzanstieg gewertet werden kann. Ob wir deshalb bei ambulanten Kurznarkosen völlig auf eine Prämedikation mit Atropin verzichten können, bleibt einer Diskussion vorbehalten.

Schwieriger ist der meist deutlich vorhandene Abfall des systolischen Blutdruckes zu interpretieren. Diese Wirkung ist wohl weniger mit einer Myokarddepression, als mit einer Herabsetzung des peripheren Widerstandes zu erklären. Vielleicht bilden sich deshalb die Blutdruckveränderungsrungen im Gegensatz zu denen des Pulses auch nur zögernd aus und erreichen erst nach einigen Minuten und auch dann nur annähernd wieder ihre Ausgangslage.

Zusammenfassung

Abschließend läßt sich zu den Ergebnissen unserer Untersuchungen folgendes sagen: Wir stimmen mit allen Autoren überein, daß Methohexital während der Narkose keine EKG-Veränderungen verursacht. Die in unseren Messungen nahezu immer aufgetretene Senkung des systolischen Blutdruckes erklären wir uns mit der Herabsetzung des peripheren Widerstandes durch eine Weiterstellung der Gefäße.

Die häufig beobachtete Zunahme der Pulsfrequenz dürfte auch unseres Erachtens auf der parasympathikolytischen Wirkung des Methohexitals beruhen.

Summary

In concluding we can comment as follows on the result of our studies: We agree with all authors concerned that methohexital does not produce any alterations in the E.C.G. during anaesthesia. The drop in the systolic blood pressure observed in almost all our measurements is explained by the reduction of the peripheral resistance due to a dilatation of the vessels.

We, too, believe that the frequently observed rise in the pulse-rate is due to the parasympatholytic activity of methohexital.

Literatur

Dundee, John W.: Charakteristika bei intraven. Narkoseeinleitung. Anaesthesist 11, 272–276 (1962).

Dundee, John W., M.D., Ph.D., F.F.A.R.C.S., Moore, James, M.B., B.Ch., F.F.A.R.C.S.: Thiopentone and methohexital. Anaesthesia 16, No. 1 (1961).

Elliott, C. J. R., Green, R., Howells, T. H.: Recovery after intravenous barbiturate Anaesthesia. The Lancet, July 14, 68 (1962).

Körner, M.: Vergleichende Beobachtungen bei verschiedenen Narkotica für die Narkoseeinleitung zur Tonsillektomie bei Kindern. Anaesthesist 14, (1965).

Lyon, Leonard Z.: Methohexital sodium: a clinical apraisal in oral surgery. Journal of oral Surgery, Anesthesia and Hospital Dental Service 19, 475–481 (1961).

Recant, Benjamin S., D.D.S.: Methohexital Sodium. Oral Surgery, oral Medicine and oral Pathology St. Louis 13, No. 11, 1330–1342 (1960).

Weyl, Ruth, Baha Unal Y. Alper: Clinical evaluation of a new ultra-shortacting oxygen-barbiturate for intravenousa nesthesia. Surgery, Gynecology and Obstetrics 107, 588–592 (1958).

Whitwam, J. G., M.B., F.F.A.R.C.S. and J. M. Manners, M.B., D.A.: Clinical comparison of Thiopentone and Methohexitone. British Medical Journal 1, 1663–1665 (1962).

Vergleichende Untersuchungen des Brenzkatechinaminspiegels bei der Anwendung von Methohexital und Thiopental

Von **R. Roggenkämper** und **I. Wilckens**

Aus der Anaesthesie-Abteilung (Chefarzt: Dr. CH. LEHMANN)
der Chirurg. Klinik und Poliklinik (Direktor: Prof. Dr. G. MAURER)
am Klinikum rechts der Isar der Technischen Universität München

Daß die Medikamentengruppe der Barbiturate ganz allgemein auf das Vegetativum Einfluß nimmt, ist bekannt und verständlich; schließlich wurde sie entwickelt, um in eine so komplexe vegetative Funktion wie den Schlaf-Wach-Rhythmus einzugreifen.

Die parasympathikolytische Wirkung des Methohexitals, auf die schon wiederholt hingewiesen wurde, tritt so zuverlässig auf, daß sich die Frage stellt, ob sich eine parasympathikolytische Prämedikation erübrigt.

Was aber geschieht mit dem Sympathikotonus? Da wir in der Literatur keine experimentell belegte Antwort fanden, nahmen wir in zwei verschiedenen Versuchsreihen quantitative Bestimmungen des gemeinsamen Abbauproduktes von Noradrenalin und Adrenalin, der Vanillinmandelsäure, vor [6, 7].

Der Nachweis dieser Vanillinmandelsäure im Urin erwies sich in den letzten Jahren als zunehmend geeignet, den Problemkreis „sympathiko-adrenales System" aufzuschlüsseln. Nach Ansicht vieler Autoren [3, 5] ist es gerechtfertigt, von der Menge der im Urin ausgeschiedenen Vanillin-mandelsäure auf den Funktionszustand des Sympathikotonus zu schließen. Das heißt also: eine Erhöhung der Brenzkatechinamine z.B. im Stress manifestiert sich mit Sicherheit in einer erhöhten Vanillinmandelsäure-Aus-scheidung im Urin. Umgekehrt führt eine verminderte Ausschüttung der Sympathikushormone mit Sicherheit zu einem Abfall der pro Zeiteinheit ausgeschiedenen Vanillinmandelsäure.

Als Indikator für die Zuverlässigkeit und Brauchbarkeit unserer Methodik testeten wir in der gleichen Versuchsanordnung Thiopental, unter dessen Wirkung YONEMARU 1964 eine signifikant erniedrigte Konzentration der Brenzkatechinamine in der Nebennierenvene beobachtete (9).

26 junge Frauen, die sich einer Abrasio unterzogen, wurden 1 Std vor der Operation aufgefordert, die Blase zu entleeren. Von einer Prämedikation

sahen wir ab, um jede Beeinflussung des Brenzkatechinaminspiegels durch andere Präparate auszuschließen. Vor und während der Narkose mit Methohexital bzw. Thiopental infundierten wir 500 ml 5,7%ige Glukose-lösung. Zur Betäubung selbst gaben wir 15 Patienten 4 mg/kg Körper-gewicht Methohexital und 11 Patienten 6 mg/kg Körpergewicht Thio-pental.

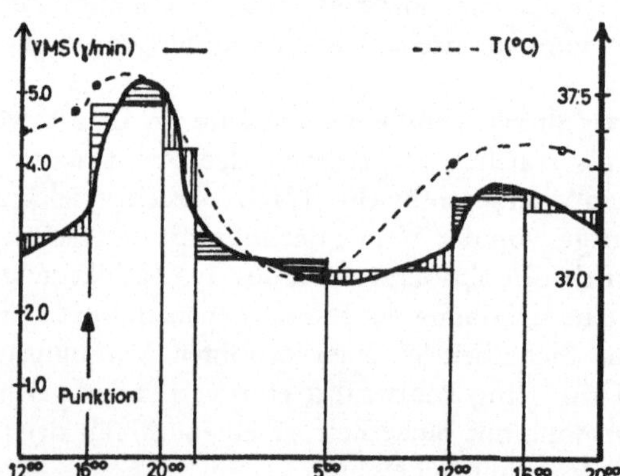

Abb. 1. Die Abszisse stellt die Zeit dar, die Ordinaten bezeichnen die gemessenen Parameter, also Vanillinmandelsäureausscheidung in γ/min, Rektaltemperatur in °C, Blutdruck und Puls

Abb. 2. Die Abszisse stellt die Zeit dar, die Ordinaten bezeichnen die beiden Parameter Vanillinmandelsäureausscheidung (γ/min) und Körpertemperatur (°C). Die Kurven demonstrieren den Verlauf von Temperatur ---- und Vanillin-mandelsäure —— über 32 Std (Mittelwerte von 21 Patienten). Die Korrelation zwischen beiden Größen ist charakterisiert durch $Y = 3{,}1545\ x\ -114{,}38$; $\nu = 0{,}74$, statistisch gesichert mit $p < 0{,}0025$

Zu Beginn der Narkose wurde ein Dauerkatheter eingeführt, der entgegen unserer ursprünglichen Planung während der Abrasio liegenbleiben mußte, weil in dem Zeitraum zwischen Narkose- und Operationsbeginn, der etwa 10 min betrug, zu wenig Urin ausgeschieden wurde.

Während dieser Zeit kontrollierten wir in Abständen von 2 min Blutdruck, Puls, EKG und die rektal fortlaufend gemessene Körpertemperatur.

Die Temperaturmessung sollte einen ersten Eindruck über Veränderungen des Brenzkatechinaminspiegels vermitteln, da zwischen diesen beiden Größen in physiologischen Bereichen eine strenge Korrelation besteht.

Aus der Betrachtung des Temperaturverhaltens ergab sich, daß die Fragestellung berechtigt und sinnvoll war.

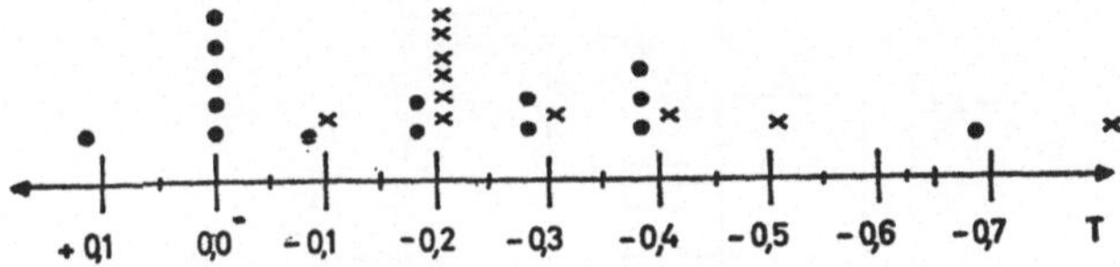

Abb. 3. Die Abszisse zeigt die Abnahme der Körpertemperatur in °C. ● bezeichnet Patienten, die Methohexital erhielten, × bezeichnet Patienten, die Thiopental erhielten. Der mittlere Temperaturabfall unter Thiopental betrug 0,3° C, unter Methohexital 0,19° C. In beiden Fällen war die Abnahme der Körpertemperatur signifikant mit $p < 0{,}0025$

Die Körpertemperatur fiel also während beider Betäubungen – unter Thiopental stärker als unter Methohexital – ab. Aus den genau protokollierten Sammelzeiten, Volumina und Urinanalysen dagegen ergab sich ein signifikanter Anstieg der Vanillinmandelsäureausscheidung pro Minute gegenüber der pränarkotischen Phase, der sicher nicht mit der Wirkung der Präparate Methohexital und Thiopental zusammenhängt, sondern einfach als Operationsstress zu verstehen ist.

Daß im Stress die Ausschüttung von Brenzkatechinaminen umgehend und erheblich erhöht wird, ist bekannt [1, 4]. Ich darf in diesem Zusammenhang an das Prinzip des Lügendetektors erinnern: hier werden innerhalb von Sekunden sympathikotone Reaktionen wie Erhöhung der Herzfrequenz und Änderung der Leitfähigkeit der Haut durch vermehrte Schweißsekretion registriert, wenn man den „Prüfling" durch die betreffende Frage in einen psychischen Stress versetzt. Daß sich aber diese Alarmreaktion des sympathikoadrenalen Systems schon 10–15 min später als Vanillinmandelsäure-Anstieg im Urin manifestiert, haben wir aus dem an sich unvorhergesehenen Ergebnis unserer ersten Versuchsordnung entnommen. Wir hatten die Geschwindigkeit des Ablaufes von Metabolismus und Ausscheidung als Vanillinmandelsäure also erheblich unterschätzt und mußten unsere Versuchsanordnung ändern.

Das geschah in der Weise, daß wir 15 Studenten, über deren Kreislaufverhalten unter Methohexital bzw. Thiopental Sie bereits von Frau Hartung
hörten, als Probanden verwandten. Bei den Untersuchungen verabreichten
wir Methohexital in einer Dosierung von 1,5 mg/kg Körpergewicht,
Thiopental in einer Dosierung von 3,75 mg/kg Körpergewicht. Die Studenten sammelten Spontanurin in zwei Portionen. Die erste stammte aus
der pränarkotischen Phase, die zweite aus dem Zeitabschnitt während und
nach der Narkose.

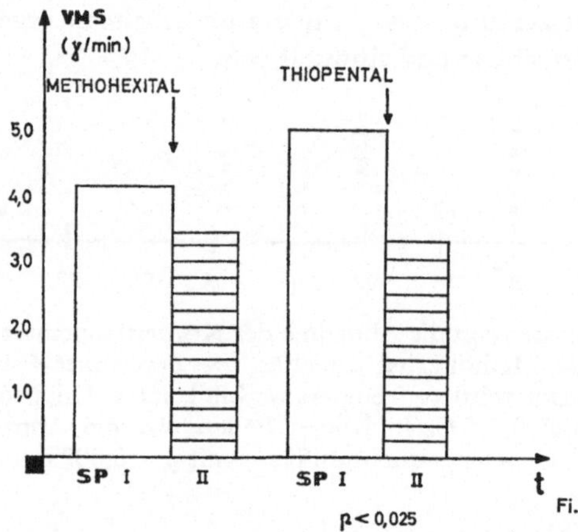

Abb. 4. Die Abszisse kennzeichnet die Zeit, die Ordinate die Vanillinmandelsäure-Ausscheidung pro Minute. Die Säulen stellen die mittlere Vanillinmandelsäure-Ausscheidung während der einzelnen Sammelperioden dar. SP I = Sammelperiode I (pränarkotisch), SP II = Sammelperiode II (intra- und post-
narkotisch). Der Unterschied zwischen den beiden pränarkotischen Werten ist
statistisch nicht signifikant. Ebenso ist der unter Methohexital beobachtete Abfall
der Vanillinmandelsäure/min nicht statistisch gesichert. Die Differenz SP I–SP II
unter Thiopental dagegen ist mit p <0,025 nicht zufällig

Die genauen Zeiten und Volumina wurden protokolliert, so daß aus
Volumen, Zeitspanne und Konzentration, die gemittelten Doppelbestim-
mungen entnommen wurden, die pro Minute ausgeschiedene Vanillinmandelsäure-Menge berechnet werden konnte (Methodik nach [2]).

Dabei ergab sich, daß unter Thiopental eine signifikante Verminderung
der Vanillinmandelsäure-Ausscheidung pro Minute erfolgte. Sie betrug
35% ± 15% und war statistisch mit 2,5% Irrtumswahrscheinlichkeit
gesichert. Unter Methohexital kam es ebenfalls zu einer leichten Erniedri-
gung, die sich statistisch jedoch nicht sichern ließ. Dieser Abfall kann
zufallsbedingt sein. Für wahrscheinlicher halten wir, daß Methohexital
im Verhältnis zu Thiopental einen wesentlich kleineren Abfall verursacht.

Diese Annahme deckt sich völlig mit den klinischen Untersuchungen, also z.B. mit denen der Temperaturveränderungen. Ein Temperaturabfall war auch unter Methohexital zu beobachten, doch war er – genauso wie die Veränderung der Vanillinmandelsäure-Ausscheidung – niedriger als unter Thiopental.

Zusammenfassung

An 26 Patienten und 15 Studenten wurde die Reaktion des sympathiko-adrenalen Systems auf die Gabe von Methohexital und Thiopental untersucht. Als Maß für den Funktionszustand des Sympathikotonus betrachteten wir – nach Schmid und Crout [3, 5] gerechtfertigt – die pro Minute ausgeschiedene Vanillinmandelsäure-Menge.

Dabei ergab sich für die 26 Patienten ein signifikanter Anstieg der Vanillinmandelsäure pro Minute, der mit Sicherheit nicht als spezifische Präparatwirkung, sondern als Reaktion auf die inzwischen einsetzende Operation zu werten ist. Wir erwähnen dies Ergebnis deshalb, weil es einen Hinweis auf die Geschwindigkeit des Mechanismus Ausschüttung–Metabolismus–Ausscheidung der Katecholamine gibt. Die Erhöhung der Brenzkatechinamine im Stress manifestierte sich bereits 10–15 min später in einer signifikanten Erhöhung der Vanillinmandelsäure-Ausscheidung.

Die bei Grundumsatzbedingungen untersuchten 15 Studenten zeigten unter der Wirkung von Methohexital einen geringen, nicht signifikanten Abfall der Vanillinmandelsäure-Ausscheidung pro Minute, während unter den gleichen Bedingungen bei denselben Studenten eine Woche später nach Thiopentalgabe die Vanillinmandelsäure-Ausscheidung pro Minute um 35% ± 15% abnahm. Dies Ergebnis ist mit 2,5% Irrtumswahrscheinlichkeit gesichert. Wir schließen daraus im Zusammenhang mit unseren klinischen Beobachtungen (Temperaturveränderungen), daß die Wirkung auf das Vegetativum bei Thiopental im wesentlichen in einer Sympathikolyse zu sehen ist, während unter Methohexital offenbar die Parasympathikolyse im Vordergrund steht. Eine statistisch signifikante Veränderung des Sympathikotonus war unter Methohexital nicht zu beobachten.

Besonderen Dank für die bei dieser Arbeit gewährte Hilfe schulden wir Herrn Prof. Lange, Herrn Dipl. Math. Reiter und Herrn Dipl. Math. Jurksch aus dem Institut für medizinische Datenverarbeitung München. Ebenso möchten wir den Kollegen von der Frauenklinik und allen beteiligten Schwestern für ihre verständnisvolle Mitarbeit danken.

Summary

The response of the sympathoadrenal system to administration of methohexital and thiopental was examined in 26 patients and 15 university students. According to Schmid and Crout [3, 5], the amount of vanilmandelic acid excreted per minute was taken as a measure for the state of the sympathotonic functions.

A significant rise in the excretion per minute of vanilmandelic acid was found to occur in all of the 26 patients. This may definitely be regarded not as an effect of the preparation per se, but the response to the intervention which in the meantime had been started. We mention this result since it demonstrates the rapidity of the mechanism release – metabolism – excretion, of the catecholamines. The rise in the pyrocatecholamine levels under stress was manifested by a significant rise in the excretion of vanilmandelic acid already after 10 minutes. Under the effect of methohexital, the 15 students examined under basal-metabolic conditions showed a low, non-significant drop in the excretion of vanilmandelic acid per minute, while, one week later, and under equal conditions, the excretion of vanilmandelic acid in the same students decreased by $35\% \pm 15\%$ following a dose of thiopental. This findings is established statistically, the probability of error being $2,5\%$. From these results and from our clinical observations (alterations in the temperatures) we conclude that the action of thiopental on the autonomic nervous system expresses itself mainly as a sympatholytic effect, while methohexital predominantly produces a parasympatholytic effect. Under methohexital, no statistically significant alterations in the sympathotonic condition were observed.

Literatur

1. CANNON, W. B.: Die Notfallsfunktion des sympathikoadrenalen Systems. Ergebn. Physiol. **27**, 380 (1928).
2. CONNELIAN, T. P., GODFREY, J. M.: The Routine Determination of Urinary 4- hydroxy- 3- methoxy-mandelic acid. Clin. Chim. Acta **9**, 410 (1964).
3. CROUT, J. R.: Sampling and Analysis of Catecholamines and Metabolites. Anesthesiology **29**, 661–669 (1968).
4. OZDIL, T., POWELL, W. F.: Urinary Output of Adrenaline and Noradrenaline during Anesthesia and Surgery: Preliminary Study. Canad. Anesth. Soc. J. **13**, 48 (1966).
5. SCHMID, E. u. Mitarb.: Untersuchungen über Physiologie und Pathophysiologie des sympathikoadrenalen Systems durch Bestimmung der VMS-Ausscheidung im Harn mit dünnschichtchromatographischer Technik. Arch. f. Kreislauff. **49**, 83 (1966).
6. SPRIGGS, T. L. B.: The Effects pf Anesthesia induced by Urethane or Phenobarbitone upon the Distribution of Peripheral Catecholamines in the Rat. Brit. J. Pharmacol. **24**, 752 (1965).
7. TSUNG HAN Li a. o.: Decreased Adrenal Venous Catecholamine Concentrations during Methoxyflurane Anesthesia. Anesthesiology **29**, 1145 (1968).
8. VOGT, M.: Effect of Drugs on Metabolism of Catecholamines in the Brain. Med. Bull. **21**, 57 (1965).
9. YONEMARU, T.: The Effects of General Anesthesia on the Catecholamine Output of the Adrenal Medulla (Japanese). Fukuoka Acta Med. **55**, 825 (1964).

Diskussion

Frey: Ich schlage vor, die ersten fünf Vorträge, die die pharmakologischen und experimentellen Grundlagen der Anästhesie mit Kurz- oder Ultrakurznarkotika behandeln, zu diskutieren.

Wer hat Fragen zum Vortrag von Herrn WHITWAM, also zur Pharmakologie des Methohexital?

Langrehr: Herr WHITWAM, ich hätte eine Frage zur intramuskulären Injektion. Ist es möglich, eine höher konzentrierte Lösung als die 1%ige zu geben? Bei der intramuskulären Verabreichung müßten wir 5–10 ml, also eine große Menge der Flüssigkeit injizieren. Kann man Methohexital in höherer Konzentration als in 1%iger Lösung verabreichen?

Whitwam: Es befaßten sich verschiedene Arbeiten mit der intramuskulären Methohexital-Verabreichung. Die allgemein empfohlene Konzentration ist die 2%ige in Kochsalzlösung. Die von MILLER empfohlene Dosis ist 6,6 mg/kg Körpergewicht. RULE vom Eastman Dental Institute und seine Mitarbeiter sowie GOLDMAN verwendeten das Mittel bei Kindern in 2%iger Lösung, und zwar ebenfalls in einer Menge von 6,6 mg/kg Körpergewicht.

Frey: Ich danke Ihnen, Herr WHITWAM. Wer hat Fragen zum Vortrag von Frau SOGA?

Zindler: Ich habe eine kurze Bemerkung zum Referat WHITWAM. Es berührt das Problem der Vergleiche. Herr WHITWAM zeigte ein Bild aus einer Veröffentlichung unserer Abteilung, das die Atemdepression nach Propanidid darstellt und integriertes Pneumotachogramm und CO_2 der Ausatmungsluft wiedergibt. Er verglich die Anordnung mit einer Methode, die die mechanische Bewegung des Thorax registriert. Diese beiden Anordnungen sind im Grunde genommen nicht vergleichbar.

Hier liegt ein Hauptproblem unserer Tagungen. Wie ist es möglich, einen gültigen Vergleich anzustellen? Das betrifft, glaube ich, auch die Ausführungen von Frau SOGA. Wir wissen, daß die Kreislaufwirkungen von Propanidid beim Hund wesentlich stärker sind und das Präparat hier ungünstig abschneidet. Deshalb ist es interessant, daß Frau SOGA jetzt auch über Untersuchungen am Menschen berichten kann.

Zum Vortrag von Frau SOGA hätte ich einige Fragen. Wurde der Katheter im linken Ventrikel in Narkose oder beim wachen Patienten gelegt? Wie weit sind die Ausgangswerte in den verschiedenen Gruppen vergleichbar und wie groß sind diese Gruppen? Frau SOGA zeigte auf ihren Bildern, was ja auch üblich und legitim ist, vom Ausgangswert ausgehende prozentuale Veränderungen.

Daß dies schwierig sein kann, beweisen die letzten Ausführungen von Frau ROGGENKÄMPER. Sie zeigte unterschiedliche Ausgangswerte der Vanillinmandelsäure bei Thiopental und Methohexital. Während der Narkose waren diese Werte gleich, so daß man sich fragen muß, wie weit die Ausgangswerte vergleichbar sind.

Dann noch eine weitere Frage. Bei dem Versuch, ein Maß für die Kontraktilität zu erhalten, das unabhängig von anderen Parametern, z.B. preload und afterload ist, führte Frau SOGA den Index von VERAGUT und KRAYENBÜHL an. Wie weit ist jedoch bewiesen und anerkannt, daß dies ein verhältnismäßig unabhängiger Parameter ist? Im übrigen sagte Frau SOGA, soweit ich mich entsinne, daß sie das Herz-Zeit-Volumen bestimmt habe, nannte aber keine Werte. Haben Sie für diese beiden Gruppen Daten zur Hand?

Soga: Nein.

Frey: Zunächst darf ich Herrn WHITWAM bitten, zu antworten.

Whitwam: Herr ZINDLER, Ihre Aufzeichnungen geben nicht nur die Kohlendioxyd-Konzentration, sondern auch das Gesamtvolumen an. Auf dem betreffenden Symposion ging aus dem vorangegangenen Vortrag von Dr. HOWELLS, dessen Manuskript ich vor mir liegen habe, ebenfalls hervor, daß das Atemvolumen, ausgedrückt in Litern pro Minute, nach der Verabreichung von Propanidid bis zu einer halben Minute lang auf Null abfiel. Ich will damit keineswegs sagen, daß Methohexital in dieser Hinsicht besser oder schlechter als Propanidid wirkt, sondern wollte lediglich betonen, daß dies meiner eigenen Erfahrung nach bei unstimulierten Patienten oft vorkommt. Wenn Sie eine Narkose im Zahnarztstuhl einleiten und unmittelbar darauf Zähne extrahieren, werden Sie damit die Atmung wieder in Gang setzen.

Daher hat der Ausdruck „Apnoe" keine Gültigkeit. Nach der respiratorischen Exzitation sieht man sowohl bei Propanidid als auch bei den Barbituraten eine Phase des „Nichtatmens". Hier tritt der Umstand ein, daß es – gleichgültig wie der Patient anästhesiert wurde – während einer Einleitung zu Phasen kommt, in denen der Patient den Atem anhält und eine Apnoe bis zu einer halben Minute zeigt. Deshalb glaube ich nicht, daß es bei der Anwendung intravenöser Narkotika irgendwelche Ausnahmen gibt. Meiner Ansicht nach treten – gleichgültig wie ein Patient vom Bewußtsein in die Anästhesie übergeführt wurde – immer Phasen der Apnoe auf. Wahrscheinlich sind diesbezüglich viele Arzneimittel vergleichbar. Es ist lediglich eine Frage, ob eine spezifische Atemdepression als Teil einer unspezifischen Einleitung von Narkosen besteht.

Frey: Danke, Herr WHITWAM. Frau SOGA, wollen Sie antworten?

Soga: Die erste Frage lautete, auf welche Weise der Kathetertipmanometer in die linke Herzkammer gelegt wurde. Wir applizierten ihn sowohl bei den Versuchstieren, als auch bei den Patienten in Lachgasanalgesie. Die Hunde wurden vorher prämediziert, relaxiert, intubiert und mit einem Lachgas-Sauserstoff-Gasgemisch kontrolliert beatmet. Zwischen dieser sogenannten Narkoseeinleitung und dem Beginn der Messung, also der Aufnahme der Kontrollwerte vergingen mindestens 1–1½ Std. Bei den Patienten leiteten wir die Narkose mit Lachgas ein. Wenn sie schliefen, wurden sie relaxiert und intubiert. Zwischen dieser Narkoseeinleitung und der Aufnahme von Kontrollwerten verging mindestens 1 Std.

Die zweite Frage lautete, inwieweit die Ausgangswerte für die geprüften Narkotika vergleichbar seien. Ich habe leider keine Tabelle dabei, die die Werte der Patienten aufzeigt, sie wird gerade angefertigt. Die Unterschiede der Ausgangswerte waren für keinen der Kreislaufparameter groß. Einige Zahlen kann ich aus der Erinnerung anführen. Der Blutdruck zum Beispeil betrug sowohl bei den Propanidid – als auch bei den Methohexital-Untersuchungen bei den Patienten systolisch 120 bis 130, diastolisch 80 bis 90. Das gleiche galt für die anderen Kreislaufparameter und den Kontraktilitäsindex.

Zu der dritten Frage, ob dieser von uns angewandte Kontraktilitätsindex repräsentativ sei und ob man die Möglichkeit habe, mit ihm Änderungen der Myokardkontraktilität exakt zu erfassen, ist folgendes zu sagen:

Der von uns benützte Kontraktilitätsindex basiert auf langjährigen Arbeiten von SONNENBLICK, SIEGEL und BRAUNWALD. Sie zeigten, daß in der isometrischen Anordnung die Änderungen der Kontraktilität am Papillarmuskel am besten mit der maximalen Kraftanstiegsgeschwindigkeit dp/dt max. wiedergegeben werden. Beim Herzen in vitro entspricht diese Größe der maximalen intraventrikulären Druckanstiegsgeschwindigkeit. Es galt nun, diesen Parameter in vivo von der enddiastolischen Ventrikelfüllung, also dem preload unabhängig zu machen. Den genannten Autoren gelang es, einen Index aufzustellen, der diese Forderung erfüllt.

Der von uns verwendete Kontraktilitätsindex nach VERAGUT und KRAYENBÜHL stellt lediglich eine technische Vereinfachung des ursprünglichen Index von SIEGEL und SONNENBLICK dar. VERAGUT und KRAYENBÜHL haben in zahlreichen Untersuchungen die Aussagekraft dieses Kontraktilitätsindexes in vivo bewiesen. Sie konnten z. B. in Untersuchungen an Hunden zeigen, daß auch bei excessiver Änderung der enddiastolischen Ventrikelfüllung durch Entbluten und massive Infusion der von ihnen vorgeschlagene Kontraktilitätsindex keine Änderung erfuhr.

Zur letzten Frage: Eine Tabelle mit den Herzzeitvolumenwerten der Patienten habe ich leider nicht hier.

Lawin: Ich habe noch eine Frage an Frau SOGA. Wie wurden die Hunde prämediziert?

Soga: Sie wurden mit einem Prämedikationsmittel, das in der Veterinärmedizin verwendet wird, nämlich mit 0,05 mg/kg Körpergewicht Kombelen prämediziert.

Lawin: Spielt bei der Vorstellung vom Abfall des peripheren Widerstandes bei Methohexital u. U. das Histamin eine Rolle, wie es vor kurzem beim Epontol nachgewiesen wurde?

Soga: Wenn diese Frage an mich gerichtet war, muß ich Ihnen sagen, daß – soweit mir bekannt ist – bis jetzt keine Untersuchungen über die Histaminproduktion in der Methohexital-Narkose durchgeführt wurden.

Frey: Bestehen Fragen zum Vortrag HARTUNG? Wenn nicht, erfolgt die Diskussion zu den Vorträgen WILCKENS/ROGGENKÄMPER und ROGGENKÄMPER/WILCKENS.

Wawersik: Frau ROGGENKÄMPER, haben Sie die Meßwerte auf Normalverteilung geprüft?

Daß Sie nach Methohexital keinen Unterschied zwischen Ausgangs- und Narkosewert nachweisen konnten, könnte allein daran liegen, daß Ihre Stichprobe zu klein, bzw. Ihr Variationskoeffizient zu groß und Ihre Meßwerte nicht normal verteilt waren. Hier möchte ich außerdem noch einmal an die Worte von Herrn Professor ZINDLER erinnern. Es erscheint mir bei solchen Untersuchungen nahezu unerläßlich, daß man die Ausgangswerte mit in die Untersuchung einbezieht. Bei all diesen Dingen handelt es sich um kovariate Probleme. Man kann Differenzen – scheinbare Differenzen – unter Umständen dadurch produzieren, daß man Unterschiede in den Ausgangswerten nicht berücksichtigt. Allein die Prüfung auf Homogenität der verglichenen Kollektive führt zu relevanten Schlußfolgerungen.

Präzise Fragen an Frau ROGGENKÄMPER: 1. Wie groß war die Anzahl der Stichproben? 2. Waren die Meßwerte bei den beiden Kollektiven normal verteilt? 3. Haben Sie die Ausgangswerte miteinander verglichen und auf Homogenität, bzw. kovariat geprüft?

Roggenkämper: Zur Frage nach der Anzahl der Stichproben: Es handelt sich um 15 Studenten, die in der ersten Woche mit Methohexital und eine Woche später mit Thiopental getestet wurden.

Zur Frage der Normalverteilung: Wir haben uns natürlich nicht angemaßt, diese Frage allein zu entscheiden, weil die statistische Berechnung darauf aufbaut, sondern baten Herrn Professor LANGE vom Institut für medizinische Datenverarbeitung in München, die Resultate zu überprüfen. Herr Professor LANGE teilte unsere Meinung, bestätigte also, daß eine Normalverteilung vorläge und wir die statistische Auswertung deshalb nach der Student-Verteilung bzw. nach dem T-Test vornehmen könnten.

Die dritte Frage betraf die unterschiedlichen Ausgangswerte. Auch wir können nicht mit Sicherheit aussagen, wodurch sie bedingt waren. Es handelt sich um die gleichen Studenten, die gleichen Tageszeiten – dies spielt ja gerade bei der Bestimmung der Brenzkatechinamine eine entscheidende Rolle – und die gleichen Bedingungen, also praktisch um Grundumsatz-Bedingungen. Wir berechneten – weil uns dieses unterschiedliche Ausgangsniveau irritierte - ob der Unterschied statistisch signifikant sei. Er war es nicht.

Das einzige statistisch gesicherte Ergebnis unserer Untersuchungen war der Unterschied zwischen den prae- und postnarkotischen Werten bei Thiopentalnarkosen.

Frey: Vielen Dank, bestehen weitere Fragen?

Büch: Führten Sie in allen Fällen die gleiche Reihenfolge, d.h. erst die Versuche mit Thiopental, so, wie Sie es eben schilderten, und dann die mit Methohexital durch? Ich könnte mir als Erklärung für Ihren Befund vorstellen, daß die Probanden beim ersten Mal in eine psychische Abhängigkeit gerieten, also sich durch Sie beruhigt fühlten, im zweiten Versuch aber wußten, was sie erwartet, also ängstlicher reagierten, und infolgedessen einen erhöhten Sympathikotonus hatten.

Roggenkämper: Die Frage, was auf die Probanden zukäme und wie sie sich fühlten, wenn sie wieder erwachten, wurde beim ersten Versuch wesentlich häufiger gestellt. Damit war also der Angst--Stress bei der Narkose mit Methohexital größer zu erwarten. Sie sind offensichtlich der Ansicht, daß die Probanden, weil sie die erste Betäubung als unangenehm empfanden, vor der zweiten Narkose wesentlich mehr Angst hatten. Unseres Erachtens dagegen mußte die psychische Belastung beim ersten Mal größer erwartet werden.

Büch: Diese Probanden setzen sich den Versuchen zunächst relativ harmlos aus, weil sie nicht wissen, was ihnen bevorsteht. Das zweite Mal sind sie aufgeregter, also liegt der Sympathikotonus höher.

Roggenkämper: Sie scheinen schlechte Vorstellungen von unserer Betäubungsform zu haben. Die Studenten arbeiteten äußerst interessiert mit und erschienen beim zweiten Mal genauso gern wie beim ersten.

Just: Bei uns wurden schon vor 10 oder 15 Jahren ähnliche Versuche mit Curare durchgeführt. Ich habe in diesen Fällen festgestellt, daß die Probanden, denen man lediglich mitteilte, daß sie ein Muskelrelaxans gespritzt bekämen, und die nicht wußten, was dies bedeutet, das Ganze als relativ harmlos betrachteten. Wenn der Versuch jedoch ein zweites oder drittes Mal durchgeführt wurde, war festzustellen, daß die Reaktionen andere waren.

Hartung: Ich möchte hier Frau ROGGENKÄMPER unterstützen. Meines Erachtens ist die psychische Belastung durch die Verabfolgung von Barbituraten und Muskelrelaxantien nicht miteinander zu vergleichen. Der psychische Stress für die Studenten war minimal. Sie halfen bei den Versuchspersonen, die vor ihnen an der Reihe waren, mit viel Freude mit, ließen sich dann betäuben und setzten sich, als sie kaum wach waren, wieder für die Versuche ein. Ihr Spaß an der Sache war so groß, daß sie uns drängten sie so bald als möglich zu neuen Untersuchungen aufzufordern.

Frey: Vielen Dank, darf ich Herrn ZINDLER bitten?

Zindler: Sie alle wissen, daß die Vanillinmandelsäure-Bestimmung und ihre Interpretation sehr kompliziert ist. Wenn ich mich richtig erinnere, lagen die Ausgangswerte bei Thiopental höher als bei Methohexital (ZINDLER skizziert die Abbildung 4 des Vortrages ROGGENKÄMPER). Das an sich Interessante ist, daß die intra- und postnarkotischen Werte übereinstimmen. Und das ist, glaube ich, das Wesentliche. Die Probanden brauchen morgens nur eine Tasse Kaffee zu trinken, um die Ausgangswerte der Vanillinmandelsäure ansteigen zu lassen. Ich weiß natürlich nicht, ob sie es taten, bzw. ob Sie sie kontrollierten.

Roggenkämper: Bei uns wird vor der Narkose grundsätzlich kein Kaffee getrunken!

Zindler: Gut. Sie wissen jedoch nicht, ob sie es nicht doch taten. Das Entscheidende ist wohl, daß die Werte während der Narkose gleich waren. Das Ganze ist etwas schwierig, die Diskussion sollte abgebrochen werden.

Frey: Vielen Dank, unsere Zeit ist so weit fortgeschritten, daß wir uns beeilen müssen. Eine letzte Frage von Herrn LANGREHR.

Langrehr: Ich wollte noch etwas zu den Arrhythmien sagen. Hinsichtlich der EKG-Registrierungen ist mehrfach betont worden, daß nie Arrhythmien aufgetreten seien. In diesem Zusammenhang darf ich auf eine Bemerkung von Herrn WHITWAM über die Apnoe und die eventuell notwendig werdende Beatmung verweisen. Eine neue Arbeit von JERRY, SHARE, REDISH, FINCH und MILLER berichtet von 100 unprämedizierten Patienten in der ambulanten Zahnheilkunde, von denen 67 % dieser Behandelten, die nach der Einleitung mit Methohexital in der Dosis von 1 mg/kg Körpergewicht über die Nasenmaske Lachgas/Sauerstoff im Verhältnis 3:1 und Fluothan in einer nicht näher angegebenen Konzentration spontan atmeten, schwerste Arrhythmien aller Typen aufwiesen.

Whitwam: Ich darf zusätzlich folgendes bemerken. Sowohl bezüglich der Elektroschock-Therapie, die – Sie werden mir darin zustimmen – eine Situation großer Belastung darstellt, als auch bezüglich Zahnextraktionen gibt es Arbeiten, die definitiv nachweisen, daß bei Methohexital eine geringere Häufigkeit der Herzarrhythmien auftritt als bei Thiopental.

Propanidid geht ebenfalls mit einem relativ niedrigen Anteil von Herzarrhythmien einher. Man nimmt an, daß es durch seine lokalanästhetische Wirkung einen antiarrhythmischen Effekt hat.

Wenn man Elektrokardiogramme im Zustand oberflächlicher Narkose aufzeichnet, in der afferente, sensible Impulse das efferente sympathische Nervensystem aktivieren, eine vermehrte Herzkontraktilität aber den peripheren Widerstand steigert, wird man, glaube ich, Arrhythmien feststellen. Ich nehme aber nicht an, daß dies in einem spezifischen Zusammenhang mit irgendeinem Mittel oder irgendeiner besonderen Technik steht. Es bedeutet lediglich, daß sich der Patient in einer oberflächlichen Narkose befindet und daß – bedingt durch eine afferente Stimulierung, insbesondere durch eine Zahnextraktion – sympathische Impulse vorhanden sind. Wenn man in dieser Situation den Blutdruck mißt, findet man, daß er während einer Zahnextraktion stets hoch ansteigt, selbst wenn Halothan in kleineren Konzentrationen dazugegeben wird.

Ich betone aber nochmals, daß ich keineswegs zu behaupten versuchte, Methohexital verursache keine Atemdepression. Ich wollte nur sagen, daß alle diese Mittel eine Atemdepression auslösen, und ich bezweifle, daß man eine wesentliche Unterscheidung zwischen ihnen treffen kann.

Frey: Ich danke Ihnen, Herr WHITWAM.

Wir fahren fort und gehen zu den klinischen Referaten über. Ich bitte Frau LEHMANN aus München um ihren Bericht über 60 000 Fälle in Methohexital-Narkose.

Klinische Anwendung des Methohexital in 60 000 Fällen

Von **Ch. Lehmann**

Aus der Anaesthesie-Abteilung (Chefarzt: Dr. Ch. LEHMANN)
der Chirurg. Klinik und Poliklinik (Direktor: Prof. Dr. G. MAURER)
am Klinikum rechts der Isar der Technischen Universität München

Die Steuerbarkeit eines Narkosemittels wird durch ihre Wirkungskurve bestimmt, die die Zeitspanne vom Augenblick des Wirkungseintrittes bis zum Abklingen des Effektes umfaßt. Gute Steuerbarkeit erfordert unter anderem unmittelbaren Eintritt der chirurgischen Narkosetiefe, also völlige Toleranz gegen schmerzhafte Eingriffe und schnelle Wiederherstellung der körperlichen und geistigen Funktionen.

Das Methohexital, ein vor 16 Jahren entwickeltes, methyliertes Oxybarbiturat, überzeugt durch schnellen Wirkungseintritt und eine kurze Erholungsphase, die auch nach längerer Narkosedauer in Erscheinung tritt.

Die kurzfristige Beeinträchtigung von Reaktions-, Koordinations-, Konzentrations- und Urteilsfähigkeit stimmt, wie die Untersuchungen von DARBOVEN zeigen, in etwa mit der des Propanidid überein, dessen Anwendung jedoch, wie DOENICKE durch direkte Bestimmung des Histaminspiegels im Blut nachwies, das Risiko exzessiver Histaminfreisetzung birgt. Die dadurch erforderliche Verabreichung eines Antihistaminikums in der Prämedikation vermindert seinen Wert als Ultrakurznarkotikum erheblich. Durch Methohexital werden allergische Erscheinungsbilder wie Erythem- und Ödembildung oder Bronchospasmus nicht ausgelöst.

Das Präparat wird wegen seines spezifischen Öl-Wasser-Löslichkeitsverhältnisses nicht wie andere Barbiturate im Fettgewebe gespeichert und zeigt auch nach während eines längeren Zeitraumes verabfolgten Repetitionsdosen keine Verzögerung seiner Desaktivierung. Während die Plasma-Clearance von Thiopental 5–15 % pro Stunde beträgt, liegt die des Methohexitals bei 15–19 %.

Unsere Versuche über die Straßenverkehrsfähigkeit nach Methohexital, über die Sie anschließend informiert werden, bewießen, daß – wenn keine Beeinträchtigung durch die Prämedikation vorliegt – Reaktions- und Konzentrationsfähigkeit schon nach 30 min wiederhergestellt sind und normales psychisches Verhalten nach 90 min vorausgesetzt werden kann. Damit erscheint gesichert, daß die Wiederherstellung der Straßenfähigkeit spätestens $1^1/_2$ Std nach Beendigung der Narkose gegeben ist.

Erfahrungen bei mehr als 60000 Narkosen erlauben uns festzustellen, daß die durch Methohexital bedingten Nebenwirkungen geringfügiger und passagerer Natur sind.

Ein auch in der Literatur häufig erwähntes Charakteristikum des Präparates stellen die in der Einleitungsphase auftretenden Exzitationsphänomene dar. Der im Vordergrund stehende Singultus kann in fast allen Fällen durch Bulbusdruck unterbunden werden. Abnorme Muskelbewegungen, Tremor, Husten und Laryngospasmus kommen seltener vor und sind durch weitere Barbituratgaben, Inhalation von Lachgas und Halothan oder Verabreichung von Relaxantien zu beseitigen.

Allzu schnelle Injektionen sollten vor allem im Bereich des Handrückens wegen der dabei auftretenden Gefäßirritation im Sinne von ziehenden Schmerzen entlang der Vene vermieden werden. Eine Neigung zu Thrombosebildungen wurde nicht beobachtet.

Die relativ hohe Potenz, die je nach Autor 2,5– bis 4fach angegeben wird, erlaubt die Anwendung einer niedrigeren Konzentration, also kleinere Gesamtdosen. In der Klinik gebräuchliche Lösungen bewirken auch bei versehentlicher intraarterieller Applikation keine Defekte, weil die Entstehung der Zellgewebszerstörung von Dosierung, Konzentration und Volumen des injizierten Barbiturates abhängt.

Unserer Erfahrung nach steht das Auftreten dieser Nebenwirkungen oft mit der Injektionsgeschwindigkeit in Verbindung. Auch der Zusammenhang mit einer gewissen Diathese ist nicht auszuschließen. Eine unserer Versuchspersonen zum Beispiel, bei der es zum Singultus kam, gab an, häufig darunter zu leiden. Andere, die sowohl während der Methohexital- als auch während der Thiopental-Narkose husteten, litten an einer chronischen Bronchitis und Erkältungen.

Wie fast alle Barbiturate wird auch Methohexital durch die Leber ausgeschieden. Dies zeigten Versuche an nephrektomierten, partiell hepatektomierten bzw. durch Tetrachlorkohlenstoff lebergeschädigten Hunden.

Bei gleicher Dosierung bewirkt Methohexital eine stärkere Leberdepression als Thiopental. Die zur Durchführung einer Narkose erforderliche geringe Menge jedoch verursacht eine wesentlich unbedeutendere Belastung, da die Beeinträchtigung der Leberfunktion – unabhängig, ob ein bereits existierender Leberschaden vorliegt – im Verhältnis zu der gegebenen Barbituratdosis steht.

Weil die Niere bei der Ausscheidung des Präparates eine untergeordnete Rolle spielt, kann das Mittel auch bei Patienten mit renaler Insuffizienz angewendet werden.

Methohexital löst in der Einleitungsphase, genauso wie andere Barbiturate und Propanidid, besonders bei rascher Injektion und Hypovolämie einen Blutdruckabfall aus, über den WILCKENS in Einzelheiten berichtete.

Nach DUNDEE, der umfangreiche Untersuchungen über die Prämedikation bei intravenösen Narkosen durchführte, wird durch diesen Faktor kein Narkoticum so weitgehend beeinflußt, wie das Methohexital. Exzitatorische Effekte werden durch die Verabreichung analgetischer Substanzen weitgehend gemildert oder aufgehoben, Wirkungsstärke und -dauer des Präparates beträchtlich erhöht.

Pharmaka wie Phenothiazine, die die Schmerzschwelle herabsetzen sollen, sind nach DUNDEE zu vermeiden, weil sie das Exzitationsstadium verstärken. Die Kombination Pethidin–Scopolamin soll einen verzögernden Effekt auf die Rückkehr des Bewußtseins haben.

Die besten Ergebnisse lassen sich seiner Erfahrung nach mit Atropin-Opiat-Verbindungen erzielen. Die hypotensive Wirkung der Opiate ist nach Methohexital geringer als nach Thiobarbituraten. Im Gegensatz zu diesen kommt es bei Methohexital nach Opiat-Prämedikation nicht zu verzögertem Aufwachen, obwohl sich während der Narkose ein barbituratsparender Effekt bemerkbar macht.

Scopolamin, das wegen seiner präoperativ gut sedierenden und postoperativ antiemetischen Wirkung viel verwendete Prämedikationsmittel, erklärt DUNDEE bei Methohexitalnarkosen als kontraindiziert, weil es die exzitatorische Wirkung dieses Mittels potenziere.

Wir konnten einen solchen Effekt nicht feststellen, sondern verwenden es in der Kombination mit Morphium als Standardprämedikation.

Da Methohexital, wie ROGGENKÄMPER schon berichtete, eine ausgeprägte parasympathikolytische Wirkung besitzt, benützen wir das Präparat in allen Fällen, in denen Atropin kontraindiziert erscheint, also bei Glaukom, Tachyarrhythmie, Hyperthyreose, hoher Temperatur und schwerem Schock.

Ob die beschriebene Wirkung berechtigt, bei Kurznarkosen grundsätzlich auf die Prämedikation mit Atropin zu verzichten, bedarf einer eingehenderen Prüfung. Unseres Erachtens ergäben sich keine Nachteile. Solange jedoch sichere Anhaltspunkte fehlen, müssen wir wegen etwaiger forensischer Konsequenzen von bindenden Empfehlungen absehen.

Die durch das steile Abklingen der Methohexitalwirkung bedingte gute Steuerbarkeit verlangt eine sorgfältige Narkoseführung. Dieser Umstand wird durch gute Prämedikation und die schnelle Wirkung der Repetitionsdosen ausgeglichen. Brauchbare Anhaltspunkte zur Steuerung der Narkose sind der mit der Hand leicht zu beurteilende Anstieg des Tonus der Kinnmuskulatur, das Wiederauftreten der Lidreflexe und leichte Abwehrbewegungen. Treten diese Zeichen auf, ist eine Nachinjektion erforderlich.

Interessant war das Ergebnis unserer Aufzeichnungen von Atmungskurven, über die HARTUNG berichtete. Bei üblicher Dosierung und normaler

Injektionsgeschwindigkeit wirkt sich die Atemdepression im Mittel nur etwa 35 sec lang aus. Dies ist kürzer, als in der Literatur angegeben wird. Auch während unserer klinischen Beobachtungen sahen wir selten eine längere respiratorische Beeinträchtigung.

Tabelle 1. *Anwendung von Methohexital zur Kurznarkose, zur Narkoseeinleitung und in Risikofällen*

Abteilung	1961-1965	1966	1967	1968	1969	1970 1.1.-30.11.	insgesamt
Chirurgie		805	1747	1877	2123	2496	9048
Thoraxchirurgie		1233	1671	1691	1524	1200	7319
HNO		1140	1364	1704	1778	1973	7959
Urologie		223	442	387	651	570	2273
Neurochirurgie		352	314	262	331	646	1905
Gynäkologie und Geburtshilfe		1388	3433	3251	2866	2533	13471
Cardiologie		81	84	123	197	231	716
Röntgendiagnostik		101	235	430	578	627	1971
Insgesamt	10473	5323	9290	9725	10048	10276	55135

Von 1961 bis zum 30. 11. 1970 verwendete unsere Abteilung das Präparat in insgesamt 55135 Fällen. Davon entfielen 26785 auf Kurznarkosen und 28350 auf die Narkose-Einleitung und -Weiterführung. In weiteren 7293 Fällen der Jahre 1966–1970 wurde das Mittel in Kombination mit der Neuroleptanalgesie angewandt (s. Tab. 1, Vortrag FINK–MEYER.)

Wir verabreichen Methohexital in 1%iger Lösung. Die Normaldosis für einen Eingriff von 5 min Dauer beträgt 80 bis 120 mg. Einmalige oder wiederholte Nachinjektionen von 10–30 mg, sowie die zusätzliche Zuführung von Lachgas und Halothan oder fraktionierten Gaben von 1–2 ml Thalamonal oder 50–100 mg Pethidin ermöglichen eine anhaltende Wirkungs-Verlängerung.

Die außerordentlich rasche Erholung mit schneller Wiederkehr der Orientierungs-, Geh- und Straßenfähigkeit erlaubt auch bei alten Menschen eine baldige Entlassung ambulant Behandelter nach Hause. Über unsere Erfahrungen bei Kurznarkosen berichtet ELCHLEPP.

Seit 1966 wenden wir Methohexital zusätzlich und in zunehmendem Maße zur Narkose-Einleitung und -Aufrechterhaltung und in Risikofällen an. Wie LANDAUER und LANDAUER bestätigen, bewährte sich das Präparat wegen seiner geringen Nebenwirkungen und des fast völligen Fehlens von Kontraindikationen bei vorgeschädigten Kranken, in Schocksituationen und für ausgedehnte Eingriffe.

Zur Sectio caesarea wird seit 2 Jahren ausschließlich Methohexital verwendet. Die Gefahr der durch Übertritt des Barbiturates vom mütterlichen zum fetalen Kreislauf bedingten kindlichen Intoxikation scheint durch Methohexital, das zwar lediglich ein Molekulargewicht von 262 hat, aber in kleinsten Dosen verabfolgt werden kann, verringert zu werden. Bauer-Ehnes stellt die physiologischen Zusammenhänge und die bei uns geübte Methode ausführlich dar.

Schließlich erweist sich das Präparat auch in Kombination mit der Neuroleptanalgesie als vorteilhaft, weil es die Einleitungsphase verkürzt und den Kranken unangenehme Erinnerungen an den Intubationsvorgang erspart. Auch in den Fällen, in denen eine vorübergehende Reduzierung des Lachgasanteiles, also ein stärkeres Sauerstoffangebot erwünscht wird, läßt sich der Zeitraum durch das Präparat überbrücken. Fink und Meier berichten Einzelheiten.

Zusammenfassung

Die Abteilung verwendete Methohexital in etwa 62 000 Fällen, von denen etwa 43% auf Kurznarkosen, etwa 45% auf Narkose-Einleitungen und -Weiterführungen und etwa 12% auf die Kombination mit der Neuroleptanalgesie entfielen. Die außerordentlich rasche Erholung mit schneller Wiederkehr der Orientierungs-, Geh- und Straßen-Fähigkeit erlaubt auch bei alten Menschen eine baldige Entlassung ambulant Behandelter nach Hause. Wegen seiner geringen Nebenwirkungen und des fast völligen Fehlens von Kontraindikationen bei vorgeschädigten Kranken, ausgedehnten Eingriffen und Schocksituationen bewährt sich das Präparat auch in Risikofällen zur Narkose-Einleitung und -Weiterführung. Die Kombination mit der Neuroleptanalgesie erweist sich als vorteilhaft, weil die Einleitungsphase verkürzt wird und Erinnerungen an den Intubationsvorgang oder akustische Wahrnehmungen während des Eingriffes wegfallen. Bei dieser Methode ermöglicht Methohexital ein vorübergehendes stärkeres Sauerstoffangebot und den Verzicht auf eine unter Umständen nicht mehr zeitgerecht applizierte letzte Fentanylgabe.

Summary

In our department, methohexital was used in 62 000 cases. In 43% of these it was employed for short-anaesthesia, in approximately 45% for induction and maintenance of anaesthesia, and in about 12% in combination with neuroleptanalgesia. Owing to the extremely rapid recovery of the patient with quick return of orientation, walking capacity and street safety, it is possible to send even the elderly patient home soon after out-patient treatment. Because of its slight side effects and the almost complete absence of contraindications in predamaged patients, extensive operations and shocksituations, the drug has proved its value also for induction and maintenance of anaesthesia in high-risk cases. Combination with neuroleptanalgesia has been found to be advantageous, since this shortens the initial phase and excludes both recall of the process of intubation on acoustic perceptions experienced during the intervention. Moreover, Methohexital permits a greater transient supply of oxygen and a last administration of Fentanyl can be omitted when, owing to special circumstances, this drug cannot be given in time.

Literatur

BARRY, C. T., RENNIE, G. G., MacPHERSON, M. M.: Methohexitone Sodium in Anaesthesia for Cyctoscopy, Anaesthesia, **17**, 176 (1962).

BELLVILLE, J. W., FENNEL, P. J., MURPHY, T., HOWLAND, W. S.: The Relative Potencies of Methohexital and Thiopental, J. Pharmacol. Exp. Ther., **129**, 108 (1960).

BINKERT, E.: Vergleichende Untersuchungen über die Straßenverkehrstauglichkeit nach Thiopental- und Methohexital-Kurznarkosen, Schweiz. Med. Wschr., **91**, 1285 (1961).

BITTRICH, M. M., KANE, A. V. R., MOSHER, R. E.: Methohexital and its Effect on Liver Function Tests, Anesthesiology, **24**, 81 (1963).

BUDD, D. C., DORNETTE, W. H. L., WRIGHT, J. F.: Methohexital for Rectal Basal Narcosis, Anesth. Analg. (Cleveland), **44**, 222 (1965).

COLEMAN, J., GREEN, R. A.: Methohexital. A Short Acting Barbiturate, Anaesthesia, **15**, 411 (1960).

DOUGLAS, M. H.: A New Intravenous Barbiturate for Pediatric Anesthesia in Difficult and Handicaped Dental Patients, Anesthesiology, **13**, 686 (1960).

DUNDEE, J. W.: Alterations in Response to Somatic Pain Associated with Anaesthesia. XVI: Methohexitone, Brit. J. Anaesth., **36**, 798 (1964).

DUNDEE, J. W.: Clinical Studies of Induction Agents. VII. A Comparsion of Eight Intravenous Anaesthetics as Main Agents for a Standard Operation, Brit. J. Anaesth., **35**, 784 (1963).

DUNDEE, J. W.: Rapidly Acting Intravenous Anaesthetics, Practitioner, **187**, 811 (1961).

DUNDEE, J. W., MOORE, J.: The Effect of Scopolamine on Methohexital Anaesthesia, Anaesthesia, **16**, 194 (1961).

DUNDEE, J. W., MOORE, J.: Thiopentone and Methohexital, a Comparison as Main Anaesthetic Agents for a Standard Operation, Anaesthesia, **16**, 50 (1961).

DUNDEE, J. W., RIDING, J. E., BARRON, D. W., NICHOLL, R. M.: Some Factors Influencing the Induction Characteristics of Methohexital Anaesthesia, Brit. J. Anaesth., **33**, 296 (1961).

FRANCIS, J. G., SMITH, K. G.: General Anaesthesia for Outpatient Bronchoscopy. I. An Attempt to Reduce the Recovery Time. II. A Clinical Trial of Methohexitone, Brit. J. Dis. Chest, **56**, 186 (1962).

GREEN, R. A.: Methohexitone, Proc. Roy. Soc. Med., **56**, 373 (1963).

GREEN, R., LONG, H. A., ELLIOTT, C. R. J., HOWELLS, T. H.: A Method of Studying Recovery After Anaesthesia. A Critical Assessment of Recovery Following Methohexitone and Thiopentone Using a Complex Performance Task, Anaesthesia, **18**, 189 (1963).

Jolly, C.: Recovery Time from Methohexital Anasthesia, Brit. J. Anaesth., **32**, 576 (1960).

Körner, M.: Vergleichende Beobachtungen bei verschiedenen Narkotica für die Narkoseeinleitung zur Tonsillektomie der Kinder, Anaesthesist, **14**, 321 (1965).

Kreuscher, H., Frey, R.: Die Verkehrstüchtigkeit unter der Wirkung von Anaesthetica, Hypnotica, Analgetica und Ataractica, Arzneimittelforschung, **12**, 1056 (1962).

Loeschcke, G. C., Soga, D., Zierl, O., Beer, R.: Vergleichende Untersuchungen über die gefäßwandschädigenden Eigenschaften verschiedener intravenöser Narkosemittel, Anaesthesist, **12**, 52 (1963).

Recant, B. S.: Methohexital Sodium. Clinical Study of a New Intravenous Barbiturate Anesthetic, Oral Surg., **13**, 1330 (1960).

Schumacher, M. J.: Brevital Sodium for Basal Anesthesia in Pediatrics, J. Am. A. Nurse Anesthetists, **30**, 283 (1962).

Whitwam, J. G., Manners, J. M.: Clinical Comparison of Thiopentone and Methohexitone, Brit. Med. J., **1**, 1663 (1962).

Whitwam, J. G., Young, D. S.: Observations on Dental Anaesthesia Introduced with Methohexitone. III Blood Pressure Changes, Brit. J. Anaesth., **36**, 237 (1964).

Wyant, G. M., Zoerb, D. L.: Propanidid-A New Nonbarbiturate Intravenous Anesthetic, Canad. Anaesth. Soc. J., **12**, 569 (1965).

Zindler, M.: Intravenöse Kurznarkose für ambulante Patienten. Barbiturate (Methohexital) und Propanidid, Deutsch. Med. Wschr., **90**, 1506 (1965).

Moderne Aspekte zur Frage der Narkose durch Inhalation, Injektion oder Infusion

Von **J. Stoffregen**

Aus dem Institut für klinische Anaesthesie
(Direktor: Prof. Dr. med. J. Stoffregen) der Universität Göttingen

I. Inhalationsnarkose

Da die Narkose spätestens seit C. L. SCHLEICH eine „gesteuerte Vergiftung" ist, ist ihre tatsächliche Steuerbarkeit für die Sicherheit ein entscheidender Faktor. Neben der Wahl des Hauptnarkosemittels spielt bei dieser Frage der Zufuhrweg eine entscheidende Rolle.

Die Inhalation ist sicherlich nicht zufällig die älteste Art, dem Organismus Narkosemittel zuzuführen. Die überragende historische Position verdankt die Inhalationsnarkose ihrer relativen Ungefährlichkeit, die darin liegt, daß sie durch Änderungen in der Konzentration des Narkosemittels vom Prinzip her steuerbar ist: Wird die alveoläre Konzentration verändert, ändert sich im gleichen Moment auch die Blutkonzentration und damit die Narkosetiefe. Wie schnell, hängt von der Wahl des Narkosemittels ab. Von allen charakteristischen Unterschieden ist die Schnelligkeit der Wirkung der wichtigste.

In der Praxis werden oft Inhalationsnarkotika mit fraktionierten Barbiturat-, Dolantin-, Valium-, Thalamonal-Injektionen u.ä. kombiniert. Dadurch werden die charakteristischen Eigenschaften der Narkosemittel bzw. ihrer Zufuhrwege mehr oder weniger miteinander vermischt. Grundsätzlich kann dabei entweder das Inhalationsnarkosemittel oder aber das intravenöse Narkotikum zur Narkose-Basis gemacht werden. Diese Kombination ist dann am sinnvollsten, wenn ein träge wirkendes Injektionsnarkotikum (z.B. Neuroleptanalgetikum) mit einem rasch wirkenden Inhalationsnarkotikum (z.B. Halothan) gemeinsam verwendet wird. Aber auch die Umkehrung ist möglich, z.B. die Kombination von Penthrane mit Pentothal. Dann übernimmt das Inhalationsnarkotikum weitgehend die Basisfunktion, während die Steuerung der Narkose in erster Linie mit relativ kleinen Pentothal-Injektionen „nach Bedarf" erfolgt. Dieses zweite Kombinationsbeispiel ist das weniger gute.

II. Injektionsnarkose

„Die subjektiven Unannehmlichkeiten der Dampfinhalations-Narkosen, welche oft die Angst des Patienten vor einer Operation übertreffen, die objektiven Folgen der Reizwirkungen in den Atmungsorganen und die Behinderung durch die Narkosemaske bei Gesichtsoperationen erweckten schon früh den Wunsch nach extrapulmonalen Narkosemitteln" (Killian, noch in der Äther-Zeit 1954).

Die ersten Versuche intravenöser Narkosemittelzufuhr lassen sich bis in die frühen Jahre nach der Erfindung der Injektionsspritze durch Pravaz 1851 zurückverfolgen. Aber diese Versuche mußten, abgesehen von Hämolyse, Thrombophlebitis und ähnlichen Schwierigkeiten, solange am Dosierungsproblem scheitern, wie nicht eine dafür geeignete Substanz gefunden war, die sich, abgesehen von der Verträglichkeit, vor allem durch kurze Wirkungsdauer bei sofortigem Wirkungseintritt und durch ausreichende narkotische Breite auszeichnete. So beginnt die Geschichte der intravenösen Narkose im engeren Sinne erst 1932 mit dem von Weese im Tierversuch erfolgreich getesteten Evipan. 1933 folgte Eunarcon, 1935 Pentothal und 20 Jahre später Methohexital (Brevimytal), das seit etwa einem Jahrzehnt in die Klinik eingeführt ist.

Etwa zur gleichen Zeit debütierte Estil, das allerdings relativ bald wegen lokaler Unverträglichkeitserscheinungen, insbesondere bei versehentlicher intraarterieller Injektion, wieder aus dem Handel gezogen werden mußte. Seit 1965 schließlich gibt es Propanidid (Epontol).

Etwa ebenfalls ein Jahrzehnt alt ist die intravenöse Narkose über fraktionierte Injektion von neuroleptanalgetischen Substanzen, um die Reihe der nennenswerten Vertreter intravenöser Narkoseverfahren kurz genannt zu haben.

Von den parenteralen Zufuhrwegen ist natürlich die intravenöse Injektion die Methode der Wahl. Da hierbei die Resorption umgangen wird, ist die Wirkung auf den Organismus bald nach der Injektion abzulesen und auf diese Weise eine bessere Dosierung möglich als bei intramuskulärer oder gar subkutaner Injektion. Allerdings wird das Wirkungsmaximum auch bei i. v. Injektion nur mit gewisser Verzögerung erreicht: Zwar besteht am Ende der Injektion der höchste Blutspiegel; die vollständige Wirkung tritt jedoch erst nach Herstellung eines Fließgleichgewichtes zwischen Blut und Gewebe ein. Bei unvorsichtiger Dosierung kann dieser Umstand zu einem Nachteil der Methode werden, weil eine versehentliche Überdosierung nicht wieder rückgängig zu machen ist.

Deshalb müssen alle intravenösen Narkosemittel, wenn ihre Wirkungsdauer kürzer ist als die gewünschte, fraktioniert appliziert werden. Dabei wiederholt sich bei jeder Nachinjektion „nach Wirkung" der eben beschriebene Mechanismus: Abhängig von Frequenz und Menge der Nachinjektionen und nicht zuletzt dem gewählten Präparat kommt es außerdem zu einer kumulativen Wirkung, die bei der Überdosierung eine wesentliche Rolle spielt.

Mithin gehört zum Bild der fraktionierten i. v.-Narkose – wegen der Notwendigkeit, diese nach „Bedarf", also nach dem klinischen Verlauf zu steuern – eine gewisse Inkonstanz der Narkosetiefe als Preis, der für die Abwehr der Überdosierungsgefahr in Kauf genommen werden muß. Diese unvermeidlichen Schwankungen dennoch in einem klinisch tolerierbaren Bereich zu halten, erfordert viel Erfahrung. Beim Ungeübten dagegen entartet sie leicht zur „Schaukelnarkose", die nicht ungefährlich ist. Deshalb lag der Ausweg durchaus nahe, die einzelnen Stöße der fraktionierten i.v.-Narkose durch die Kombination mit einer Inhalationsnarkose „abzuschwächen", d.h. das Inhalationsnarkosemittel zur Narkose-„Basis" zu machen und recht und schlecht die Narkose „nach Bedarf" durch kleinere i.v.-Fraktionen zu vertiefen. Die umgekehrte Kombination (z. B. Dehydrobenzperidol und Fentanyl mit Halothan) ist allerdings vernünftiger.

III. Infusionsnarkose

Ein anderer Ausweg aus dem Schaukel-Dilemma der i.v.-Narkose bietet sich in Form der Infusionsnarkose an. Dabei wird die Infusionslösung nur noch als Vehikel für die Zufuhr des Narkosemittels verwendet. Schon in den 40er und 50er Jahren war der „Evipan-Dauertropf" ein nicht ungebräuchliches Verfahren in unseren Operationssälen, das besonders bei längerdauernden Eingriffen verwendet wurde, in der Regel allerdings kombiniert mit einer Äther-Inhalation, und nach genereller Einführung von Narkosemaschinen auch mit Lachgas und Sauerstoff. Obwohl dabei im Bedarfsfall durch Erhöhung der Infusionsgeschwindigkeit die Narkose momentan vertieft werden konnte, blieb die Evipan-Infusion doch wegen des relativ ungeeigneten Narkosemittels praktisch unsteuerbar und bedeutete keinen wesentlichen Fortschritt gegenüber der Basis-Narkose durch einen Avertin-Einlauf der 30er Jahre.

Die Renaissance der Infusionsnarkose brach erst an mit der Einführung der wirklich ultrakurzwirkenden Narkosemittel auf Injektionsbasis: Methohexital und Propanidid. Schon 1964 berichteten HARGROVE u. PEARCE [1] über Bronchoskopie-Narkosen, die sie nach Injektionseinleitung mit Methohexital mit einer intravenösen Infusion von 0,1% Methohexital in 5%igem Traubenzucker unterhielten. Allerdings kombinierten sie das Verfahren mit der Lokalanaesthesie und relativ hohen Dosen von Succinylcholin. Ebenfalls 1964 berichteten COLEMANN und DE VILLIERS [2] günstige Erfahrungen mit der intravenösen Methohexital-Infusion bei 140 Parkinson-Patienten bei stereotaktischen Eingriffen. Dabei war anfangs die

Unterdrückung des Tremors und der abnormen Bewegungen aber nur durch ungewöhnlich hohe Methohexitaldosen möglich, so daß sie später das Verfahren mit 40-50 mg Gallamin bei entsprechend verminderter Barbiturat-Konzentration befriedigend kombinierten. 1694 veröffentlichte Meagher [3] gute Resultate mit 0,1%iger Methohexital-Infusion in einer Serie von 40 Patienten mit Operationen mit dem extrakorporalen Kreislauf und fand, daß Methohexital sowohl dem Pentothal als auch dem Halothan wegen der fehlenden Kreislaufdepression und Hypotension und auch im Hinblick auf die prompte und gleichmäßige postnarkotische Erholung überlegen war.

Wangeman [4] verwendete schon 1962 mit gutem Erfolg eine 0,2%ige Methohexital-Infusion als Adjuvans für leichten, steuerbaren „Schlaf" bei Operationen in Lokalanaesthesie.

Propanidid-Infusionsnarkosen sind demgegenüber bisher nur vereinzelt berichtet worden, vorwiegend von italienischen Kollegen im Zusammenhang mit geburtshilflicher Analgesie.

Beide Substanzen, Methohexital und Propanidid, sind für die Applikation per infusionem wegen ihrer kurzen Wirkungsdauer weit eher prädestiniert als ihre Barbiturat-Vorgänger vor 20 Jahren. Trotzdem bleibt die Frage diskutabel, ob nicht die Kombination mit einer entsprechend verminderten Halothan-Inhalation ebensoviel Vorteile bietet.

IV. NLA per infusionem

Als vor einem Jahrzehnt die NLA als Narkoseverfahren praktikabel wurde, kam den neuroleptanalgetischen Substanzen der Umstand sehr entgegen, daß das konkurrierende Halothan infolge seiner raschen und starken Wirkungweise in den ersten Jahren der klinischen Einführung Überdosierungsgefahren heraufbeschwor, die zu vermeiden man erst erlernen mußte. So waren Spezialverdampfer erforderlich, neue Kenntnisse und Erfahrungen in der Kombination eines potenten Inhalationsnarkosemittels mit künstlicher Beatmung, auch mit Respiratoren usw. Deshalb kam es in der Einführungszeit von Halothan relativ oft zu Herzstillständen, die mangelnder Reanimationstechnik wegen nicht selten tödlich verliefen und die Anaesthesisten verständlicherweise sehr belasteten. Nicht wenige namhafte Kollegen warnten öffentlich vor der Halothan-Anwendung, das sie als den Versuch verteufelten, „das Chloroform quasi durch die Hintertür wieder in die moderne Anaesthesie einzuschleusen".

Dabei waren die späten 50er Jahren durchaus reif für neue Narkose-Mittel bzw. -verfahren, da die damaligen Möglichkeiten der Anaesthesie mit fraktionierten Barbituratinjektionen in Lachgas-Sauerstoff oder gar Äther mit (Teil-) Curarisierung jeden nachdenkenden Anaesthesisten geradezu zur Kritik herausfordern mußten. Es ist nur verständlich, daß die NLA ebenso wie Halothan auf ungewöhnliches Interesse stießen und von den Promotoren unseres Faches als möglicher Ausweg aus dem Dilemma hoffnungsvoll begrüßt wurden.

Den Wettlauf hat Halothan bisher mit großem Abstand gewonnen. Die Ursache für diesen an sich nicht verdienten Ausgang liegt meines Erachtens in der folgenschweren Verkennung der Steuerungsaufgaben für die NLA-Narkose. Die propagandistische Bagatellisierung des Problems mag zum Teil ihre Begründung in der Rivalität zum Halothan finden, für das die Schwierigkeit der sicheren Steuerung in den ersten Jahren fast tödlich zu werden drohte. Psychologisch schien deshalb ein möglichst großer Abstand der NLA von den Dosierungsnöten des Konkurrenten taktisch klug zu sein – und war das wohl auch für eine gewisse Zeit.

Dennoch ist die Steuerung (und damit die Steuerbarkeit) der Narkose (siehe C. L. SCHLEICH 1897) der wesentliche Punkt, in dem sich die moderne Anaesthesie von den unqualifizierten Narkosepraktiken der Vergangenheit unterscheidet.

Die um 1960 ad hoc entwickelten Dosierungsempfehlungen für NLA in Form mehr oder weniger fraktionierter intravenöser Injektionen von DHB und FE (z.B. NLA-Typ I bis III) waren primitiv und können nur als diskutabel gelten, wenn sie bei ausgewähltem Krankengut unter Beachtung bestimmter Kautelen angewendet werden. Im gleichen Maße wie Halothan seine Kinderkrankheiten verlor und „erwachsen" wurde, mußte die NLA ins Hintertreffen geraten. Nur die in der Tat ungewöhnlich gute Toleranzbreite von DHB und FE konnte (bei Inkaufnahme unnötig eingeengter Indikation und bestimmter Erschwerungen in der postnarkotischen Fürsorge des Patienten) diese Anwendungsfehler solange vertuschen. Dennoch haben die Fußangeln der fraktionierten Injektionen die NLA-Anwendung bisher so begrenzt, daß wir noch 1970 kaum weiter sind als 1962.

Erst durch die Infusion ist die NLA tatsächlich steuerbar geworden. Wir verwenden dabei folgende Technik, die sich inzwischen bei mehr als 18000 Patienten bewährt hat: Im Erwachsenenalter leiten wir die Narkose (mit oder ohne Prämedikation mit 2 ml Thalamonal und 0,5 mg Atropin) mit einer Schußinjektion von 80–100 mg Brevimytal ein, unmittelbar gefolgt von 4 (-2) mg Pancuroniumbromid, 100 mg Succinylcholin, Intubation und automatischer IPP-Beatmung mit N_2O-O_2 im Verhältnis von 2 bis 3 zu 1. Das dauert nicht mehr als 20 sec. Dann wird die Infusion mit 12,5 mg DHB und 1,0 mg FE pro 500 ml (mit einem blauen Pflaster markiert) angeschlossen, die durchschnittliche Infusionsgeschwindigkeit beträgt 25–32 Tropfen pro min. Säuglinge und Kleinkinder (etwa bis zum 6. Lebensjahr), die wir schon seit langem nicht mehr prämedizieren, erhalten eine Infusion von nur noch 10 mg DHB und 1,0 mg FE pro 500 ml (grünes Pflaster) mit einer dem Alter und der Situation entsprechenden Tropfgeschwindigkeit, die etwa zwischen 8 und 20 Tropfen pro min variiert.

Bei kleineren Kindern, denen eine Venenpunktion nicht zugemutet werden kann (obwohl wir zur Narkoseeinleitung grundsätzlich zur Vermeidung überflüssiger Katecholaminausschüttung dünne Kanülen verwenden), beginnen wir die Narkose wie auch früher mit Halothan und injizieren, sowie das Kind eben schläft, 100 mg Succinylcholin auf der Außenseite des Oberschenkels intramuskulär, intubieren etwa 30 bis 60 sec später in immer noch flacher Halothan-Narkose und beatmen danach in gleicher Weise.

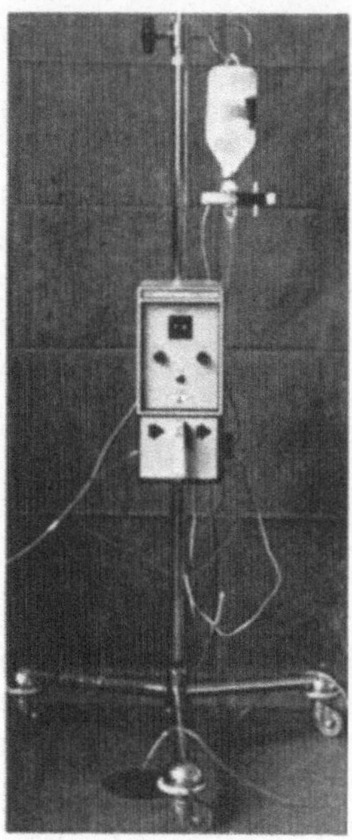

Abb. 1. Nach dem Fingerprinzip arbeitende Infusionspumpe IVAC 501 mit photoelektrischem Tropfenfühler und zwischen 1–99 wählbarer Tropfgeschwindigkeit pro min. (Lieferfirma Tekmar-Elektronik, 8 München, Oskar-Miller-Ring)

Nach der Venae sectio wird die Halothan-Zufuhr abgestellt und die entsprechende „blaue" oder „grüne" NLA-Infusion angeschlossen, die etwa im angegebenen Rahmen individuell dosiert werden muß. Außerdem erhalten die Kinder gegebenenfalls Pancuroniumbromid.

Die NLA-Narkose applizieren wir möglichst über eine Infusionsmaschine (Abb. 1), die die NLA-Infusionsnarkose nahezu so steuerbar macht wie eine Halothan-Inhalationsnarkose über den Fluotec Mark 3: Über die Änderung der mit großer Genauigkeit verabfolgten Tropfenzahl kann die NLA-Narkose in jedem Augenblick nicht nur vertieft, sondern auch verflacht werden. Wenn keine Infusionsmaschine verfügbar ist, bedeuten

Tropfenzähler (Abb. 2) eine große Hilfe, da sie aus zwei aufeinanderfolgenden Tropfen die Tropfgeschwindigkeit pro min. momentan extrapolieren. Durchschnittlich benötigen wir pro Narkosestunde eine NLA-Infusionsmenge beim Erwachsenen von 100 ml, das sind nur 2,5 mg DHB + 0,2 mg FE. Die Infusionsmengen bei kleinen Kindern mit der verringerten DHB-Konzentration sind entsprechend.

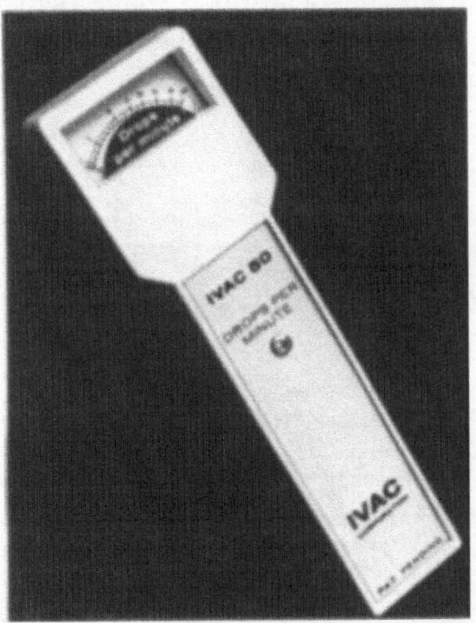

Abb. 2. Batteriebetriebener Tropfenzähler IVAC 50

Mit Hilfe der geschilderten Infusionstechnik ist es gelungen, auch die NLA wie die Halothan-Narkose „innerhalb weniger Atemzüge" steuerbar zu machen, also gegebenenfalls auch wieder zu verflachen oder zu beenden. Sie ist damit Halothan quoad Steuerbarkeit etwa ebenbürtig geworden; sie ist ihm überlegen hinsichtlich der fehlenden Ganglioplegie und weil sie mit Sicherheit auch im seltenen Ausnahmefall nicht hepatotoxisch ist. Damit umfaßt der NLA-Indikationsbereich praktisch die gesamte Anaesthesie mit wenigen Ausnahmen, wie z. B. die Einleitungsphase bei Säuglingen und Kleinkindern, denen eine Venenpunktion nicht zugemutet werden kann.

Die hinreichend bekannten (wenn auch oft bestrittenen) Nachteile von Halothan sind Myokarddepression, Plegie peripherer Ganglien (damit Einschränkung des Kreislaufregulationsapparates), schwache Analgesie (mitunter deshalb schwierige Dosierung) und die zwar seltene, aber doch im Einzelfall nicht sicher auszuschließende Möglichkeit postnarkotischen Lebersversagens (besonders bei Zwei- bzw. Mehrfachnarkosen und entsprechender „Sensibilisierung"). Seine Vorteile sind die rasche und reversible Wirkungsweise, die Kleinvolumigkeit, Unbrennbarkeit und (meist) ausgezeichnete postnarkotische Verträglichkeit. Dieselben Vorteile gelten auch für die NLA-Infusionsnarkose, aber ohne diese Nachteile.

V. Apparative Verbesserungen

Erlauben Sie mir abschließend noch einige Bemerkungen zur apparativen Seite unseres Narkosefaches: Im ketzerischen Gegensatz zur herrschenden Lehre sind wir keineswegs der Meinung, daß ein Maximum an

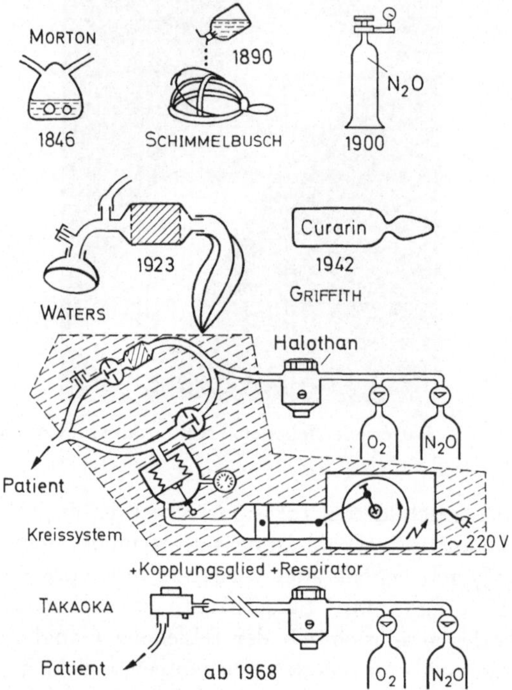

Abb. 3. Schematische Darstellung der wesentlichen apparativen Entwicklungsgeschichte der Anaesthesie. Schraffiert das obsolete Narkosekreissystem mit Kopplungsglied und Respirator (s. Text)

Maschinerie zugleich auch ein Maximum an Sicherheit für den Patienten bedeuten müßte. Vielmehr scheint es uns reichlich – und gefährlich – naiv, den Höhepunkt der apparativen Entwicklung in der mehr oder weniger historischen Aneinanderreihung der Einzelteile (Abb. 3) zu sehen, die in den letzten 100 Jahren entwickelt wurden. So halte ich die von Waters 1923 eingeführte CO_2-Filtrationsmethode nicht etwa für einen Fortschritt

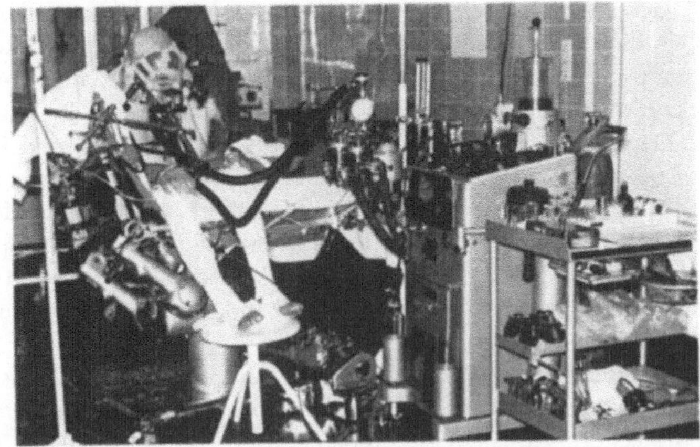

Abb. 4. „Historisches" Kreis-(Rückatmungs-)System mit Kopplungsglied und Respirator in situ

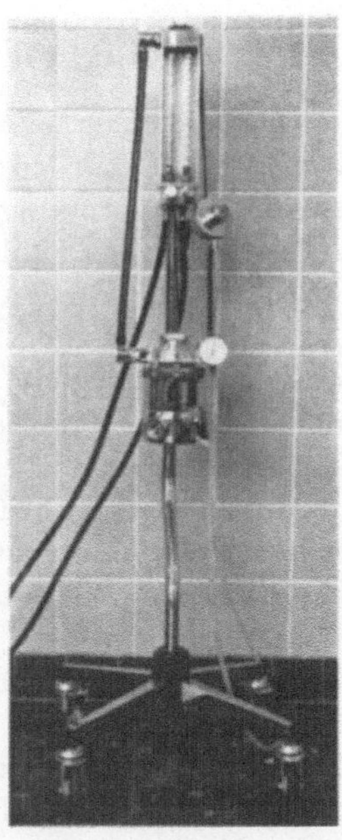

Abb. 5. Halboffenes Narkosesystem „Modell Göttingen" (Herstellerfirma BOC-Deutschland, 565 Solingen, Schulstraße 14) mit Fluotec Mark 3 und Takaoka-Respirator

unseres Faches, sondern vielmehr für einen der folgenschweren Irrtümer in der Geschichte der Anaesthesie: Es ist grotesk, den Patienten durch entsprechend komplizierte Apparaturen zu zwingen, seine eigene Ausatmungsluft rückzuatmen, die mit Hilfe eines Absorbers von CO_2 befreit wurde. Es wäre genauso unsinnig, wenn wir beispielsweise Auspuff und Vergaser unserer Autos über einen (Falten-)Schlauch miteinander verbinden wollten.

Das Rückatmungssystem hat keine Vorteile, dafür aber immense Nachteile, weil es ebenso kostspielig wie aufwendig ist, fehleranfällig und wartungsbedürftig. Allein die Unübersichtlichkeit solcher Monstren (Abb. 4) ist nicht selten Ursache tödlicher Komplikationen gewesen – quod erat demonstrandum.

Stattdessen scheint es uns vernünftiger, ein halboffenes Narkosesystem zu verwenden, das wir direkt über den Takaoka-Respirator mit dem Endotrachealtubus des Patienten verbinden (Abb. 5). Nicht zuletzt deshalb, *um das fehleranfällige und lebensgefährliche Rückatmungssystem zu vermeiden*, wurden in Göttingen in den letzten Jahren z.B. alle Patienten, die mit dem extrakorporalen Kreislauf operiert werden mußten, mit Takaoka-Respiratoren beatmet. (Saint-Exupéry: „Fortschritt heißt, das unvollkommen Komplizierte vollkommen unkompliziert zu machen.")

VI. Methohexital

Zum Schluß lassen Sie mich – nicht nur aus Höflichkeit – zum Methohexital zurückkehren: Nach den Enttäuschungen mit Propanidid, das bei uns in einer relativen Häufigkeit von einer auf weniger als 1000 Narkoseeinleitungen zum Herzstillstand führte, vielleicht infolge massiver Histaminliberation (darüber haben wir u.a. auf dem Straßburger Kongreß berichtet), verwenden wir etwa vom 4. Lebensjahr an zur Narkoseeinleitung nur noch Methohexital, und zwar als zügige Injektion von 1–1,3 mg pro kg Körpergewicht und unabhängig davon, ob die Narkose anschließend mit Halothan oder einer NLA-Infusion unterhalten werden soll.

Die erhofften günstigen Erwartungen haben sich bei Risikopatienten ebenso bestätigt wie bei 450 Patienten in der offenen Herzchirurgie einschließlich 64 Herzklappenersatzoperationen, bei mehr als 80 Kaiserschnittentbindungen, bei Defibrillationen, mehr als 400 Elektroschockbehandlungen in der Psychiatrie, bei Asthmatikern und in der ambulaten Praxis.

Unbefriedigend dagegen sind unsere Erfahrungen bei 20 Patienten gewesen, die wir unter 0,1%iger Methohexital-Infusion bronchoskopiert haben, weil es nicht gelang, den Hustenreiz ohne Lokalanaesthesie-Zusatz ausreichend zu unterdrücken. Ob das mit einer 0,2%igen Infusion unter Addition von 0,5 mg Fentanyl gelingt, bleibt abzuwarten.

Zusammenfassung

Insgesamt darf ich unsere Methohexital-Erfahrungen so zusammenfassen, daß dieses intravenöse „Narkotikum" wegen seiner kurzen Wirkungsdauer und der fehlenden Nebenwirkungen auf angenehmste Weise seinen Barbituratursprung verleugnet. Es ist dem Propanidid überlegen und erfüllt zum ersten Mal die Ansprüche, die optimistische Anaesthesisten sich schon von der Evipan-Einführung vor vier Jahrzehnten erhofften.

Summary

Summing up our experiences with methohexital, I may say that this intravenous anaesthetic disowns its origin as a barbiturate in a very pleasant manner for the duration of its action is short and it lacks untoward side-effects. Methohexital proved superior to propanidide and would seem to be the first anaesthetic to fulfill the hopes optimistic anaesthesists have been expressing even before the advent of Evipan four decades ago.

Literatur

1. HARGROVE, R. L., PEARCE, D. J.: Anaesthesia **19**, 226 (1964).
2. COLEMAN, D. J., DE VILLIERS, J. C.: Anaesthesia **19**, 60 (1964).
3. MEAGHER, R. P.: Curr. Res. Anaesth. **43**, 679 (1964).
4. WANGEMAN, C. P.: Curr. Res. Anaesth. **41**, 307 (1962).

Brietal Sodium as an Induction and Maintenance Agent

By **D. J. Coleman**

St. Georges Hospital Group, London
The National Hospital for Nervous Diseases, London
The Royal Masonic Hospital, London, England

In any field of work, progress and change go hand in hand. Induction of anaesthesia has become associated with the name thiopentone – and frequently the very term anaesthesia suggests thiopentone. Up to a point this is fair, for thiopentone has been an exceedingly useful anaesthetic tool. However this whole imagery of anaesthesia and thiopentone is the first major misconception that besets every student taking his initial shaky step into the polyglot world of anaesthetic pharmacology; i.e. the assumption that anaesthesia is synonymous with narcosis. Today this is simply not true. We are concerned with the induction of sleep, not, I stress, narcosis – and in some instances merely with inducing a state of unawareness. Thus with this change of emphasis on the role of the induction agent it necessarily followed that a search was made for drugs with pharmacological actions more suited to the conception of "induction".

The discovery, development and availability of such new drugs has meant not only a change of established and well-tried methods but also the need to acquire and understand new techniques and it must be admitted that in this field – as in every walk of life – change tends to be resisted.

I submit that methohexitone has precipitated just that sort of change in anaesthesia today and I propose to explain just why and how methohexitone should be utilised in modern anaesthesia. Literature on this drug is legion and freely available and therefore I shall restrict my paper to a discussion on its practical involvement.

Since 1959 I have been advocating the use of the 1 % solution, i.e. 10 mg per ml. This solution, properly prepared, is stable for long periods – far longer than that suggested by the manufacturers. Care must be taken to ensure that the mixture is not contaminated by acidic sterilising fluids during preparation – particularly during the cleaning of the rubber stopper on the bottle; it is far better actually to remove the cap of the "Brietal" bottle and pour in the necessary volume of water or saline. "Made-up" in this way "Brietal" is non-irritant and therefore leakage back from the vene-puncture site or even from extra-venous injection is not in any way hazardous. Indeed STOELTING (V.K. 1957), gave small intra-arterial doses with little response and I have given doses of up to 100 mg of the 1 % solution intra-arterially, to anaesthetise calves, with no demonstrable effect – locally or distally. A total dosage of 100 mg of 1 % solution need never normally be exceeded for induction purposes and if you remember that a dose of this order can be given – with caution – to a 3 year old or to an 83 year old patient, then the margin of safety is apparent. However I would not advocate that doses of this order should be administered; I believe the best ratio to be 5–7 mg per stone or an average of 1 mg per kg. For some procedures a far smaller dosage can be used with effect. What is of great importance is that – except in the very old, very young or very ill – the pre-determined dose should be given as fast as possible, through a small bore needle (no. 20), as this is both kindest to the patient and allows for an adequate time/volume concentration to be injected.

"Brietal" given in this way for the induction of sleep, has little effect on the blood pressure, blood flow or capillary bed and allows adequate time for the competent anaesthetist to complete such procedures as laryngeal spray, insertion of gastric tube, oesophageal thermocouple or other monitoring devices and intubation. There is, in fact, little difference in the time available for completing these various procedures than when using equipotent dosages of thiopentone. It is unfortunate that in the same way as there developed a tendency to give more than the minimal requirement of thiopentone, there is now all too often a tendency to use methohexitone in greater concentration than is required and in larger total dosage than is strictly needed; this trend is much to be deprecated.

The minimal effect that methohexitone exhibits on the blood pressure is important – for this means that the drug can safely be used as an induction agent in a variety of difficult situations. For example, it can be used for patients in the sitting position; for hypertensive and elderly patients. In this respect "Brietal" approaches the ideal induction agent more closely than any other drug, as the drift to sleep is rapid, pleasant and free from disagreeable sensations of taste or smell.

A point worth noting is whether correct administration of "Brietal", is related to the type of premedication. Before receiving supplies of "Brietal", in company with others, I was using thiopentone in 1.25 % solution and was therefore anticipating a more concentrated drug that did not have a basal-narcotic type action: i.e. which prolonged into the maintenance period of the administration. Premedication with agents that depress respiration when given in effective premedicant dosage – and so often they are not – will emphasize this aspect of any induction agent; therefore the use of hypnotic drugs is preferable in this respect as it provides continuity of effect, from night sedation, through premedication, to induction. Thus the transition from the onset of sleep to the period of maintenance of anaesthesia, can be achieved without any break in the respiratory effort and with minimal effect on its pattern.

However, when intubation is required, the occurrence of an apnoeic period is immaterial, as the sleep dose of "Brietal" should be followed immediately by the relaxant drug and the intubation performed without inflating the lungs with oxygen. When this procedure is followed there is no change in the blood gas analysis from pre-induction until the onset of ventilation or spontaneous respiration with high oxygen concentration. This technique pre-supposes a certain proficiency in intubation and is, of course, unsuitable for teaching purposes. Inflating the lungs with air and oxygen is not, however, a major factor – nor is it of great importance at which exact point in the procedure it is performed; but it should be recognised that whenever inflation is enacted in the absence of intubation, gas is forced into the stomach, thus increasing the risk of post-operative discomfort – often manifesting as nausea – which may be subsequently cited as a complication of the drug.

From time to time reports are received that "Brietal" precipitates some form of involuntary muscle movement and it should be noted that any barbiturate drug may have this effect on some individuals – thiopentone is no exception. From my experience I must conclude that such an incidence is extremely rare as I have never experienced evidence of muscular movements in any of my own cases.

"Brietal" may be given to children both orally and rectally, but as the oral dosage is large and, however the solution disguised, must appear somewhat unpalatable and the volume required rectally is also large, these methods are unsuitable for general purposes.

It is common practice to remove false dentures before administering an anaesthetic but when giving "Brietal" by continous infusion, in a patient who is expected to be roused during the operation, it is preferable not to do so – as in such cases the dentures act as an airway and assist articulation during wakefulness thus giving the patient a measure of confidence and dignity.

Complete clinical recovery from induction doses of "Brietal" is rapid and much subsequent discussion has centred around this particular aspect of the drug. When other points already mentioned are taken into consideration with this, the drug presents as a most suitable and tempting agent for use in out-patient work – including Electro Convulsive Therapy, obstetrics, dental work and psychiatric practices such as hypnosis and abreaction.

Without doubt, rapid recovery is certainly most desirable – especially considering the purely physical difficulties of accommodation in the busy out-patient department – with E.C.T. cases and dental patients. A well trained team should have little difficulty with the E.C.T. patients. The dose of

"Brietal" is calculated from the lower ranges as the patient is often dosed with a multitude of drugs – e. g. 0.5–0.8 mg. per kg. Thus a patient weighing 12 stone (or 168 lbs or 77 kg), would receive between 40–60 mg. This induction dose is followed immediately by an appropriately small dose of succinylcholine chloride to modify the convulsive effect of the shock and the lungs may be inflated once – with 100 % oxygen before the shock is induced. Recovery is rapid and uneventful and hyperventilation with air or oxygen is contra-indicated.

The form and time of recovery show a marked difference on the same patients when managed as described above from when sleep is induced with other barbiturates. Waking from sleep is invariably rapid and calm; disorientation, confusion and excitement are noticeably absent and the patient tends to take up conscious thought from the point where sleep was induced, without appreciating that there has been an intervening period. Furthermore the unpleasant taste/smell sensations commonly noted with thiobarbiturates do not occur with "Brietal".

Induction of anaesthesia for operative obstetrics has many points in common with that required for minor out-patient surgery or dentistry, but the obstetric patient is frequently even more apprehensive than the average out-patient. Fear of the unknown; fear of death and possibly latent fears concerning the physical state of the unborn child, all play a part – but fear of pain is paramount. The woman may also have taken food, possibly in quite large amounts, only a short while before anaesthesia is required. The induction should therefore be rapid and free from further trauma and any inhalation method is contra-indicated. In these circumstances "Brietal" should be used in the same dosage as for the E.C.T. patient, followed immediately by a small dose of succinylcholine chloride, to facilitate intubation. It thus provides a smooth, rapid and pleasant induction without any fall in the blood pressure or other unwanted side-effects; it is rapidly removed from the blood stream and has no noticeable effect on the child born some minutes later. Subsequent anaesthesia is maintained with 50 % nitrous oxide and oxygen, with minimal adjuvants, such as trichlorethylene or cyclopropane.

Occasionally, pain may be experienced from the injection of "Brietal" along the path of the vein. In some instances this may be due to the spirit, or other cleanser used to prepare the skin, being carried into the vein by the point of the needle; in others, it may be that a damaged or barbed needle has lacerated the vein wall or that a rigid vein, which can be as sensitive as an artery, has been punctured. Injection of water can produce the same response. However, such pain is neither severe nor prolonged; it is not recalled by the patient and is of no real significance.

"Brietal" therefore can be recommended, either as the sole agent of choice or as an induction agent, for all in-patient and out-patient work requiring anaesthesia.

"Brietal Sodium" can also be used successfully, in certain specific cases, as a maintenance agent. Its use in these circumstances can be divided into those cases requiring single doses, which may be repeated once or twice should conditions dictate and those cases requiring continuous intravenous infusion over a lengthy period. An example of the former, is that of alcohol injection of the trigeminal sensory root for "Tic Douloureux" which when successful, produces life-long trigeminal sensory loss. Compared with any of the major trigeminal operations, it has the advantage of safety and makes hospitalisation unnecessary – with the exception of a few patients with disseminated sclerosis and a consequent paraplegia, and a very few with prolonged post-operative vertigo and vomiting.

"Brietal Sodium" was finally selected for trial in this instance because of its short duration of effect and the speed and completeness with which patients regained consciousness without drowsiness or a hangover. Moreover, the minimal effect the drug exerts on the blood pressure enables an effective dose to be administered to elderly patients who often suffer incidental cardiovascular disease. The continuance of spontaneous respirations obviates the possibility of anoxia, provided that obstruction to the airway is prevented. The average age of these patients is 64, and the oldest in my series was 88. The mean time taken to introduce 3 needles through the foramen was a little over $2^1/_2$ min (range 1–6 min). An average time of $5^1/_2$ min (range 3–8 min) was taken from the injection of "Brietal" until the patient was able to make an adequate verbal response. There was an impressive lack of residual drowsiness or hangover effect or delay due to inability of the patient to co-operate in sensory testing. The average drop in systolic blood pressure in a decidedly elderly age group was 11 %. The largest systolic drop was from 160–115 mm mercury and lasted but a few seconds, since the pressure rose to 170 mm mercury as soon as the trigeminal needle entered the foramen ovale. This return to a normal or above normal level following the application of a stimulus, is invariable. Dr. Penman and I do not consider this sequence to be any more dangerous than the fall of pressure which occurs when the normal subject stands up from a lying position.

The site of skin puncture lies in the lower cheek which necessitates the use of a nasal mask if inhalation anaesthesia is employed and even this kind of mask comes awkwardly near to the trigeminal needles. While the needles are being aimed and passed, the patient's head has to be raised moderately and his neck somewhat flexed. If the tips of the needles are in Meckel's Cavity and well separated, one of the needles must be inserted as far laterally as possible on this cheek; this is incompatible with forced protrusion and over-closure of the lower jaw, which would bring the coronoid process of the mandible forward into the path of the lateral needle. These two requirements may lead to difficulties in maintaining a satisfactory airway but the duration of anaesthesia only amounts to a few minutes. A further 10 min are spent in taking and developing radiograms after which the patient must be capable of describing accurately the sensations induced by the injection of alcohol and of co-operating intelligently in sensory testing.

Therefore an essential part of trigeminal sensory root injection is the passage of a needle – and often several needles – through the foramen ovale. This is usually very painful unless it can be covered by general anaesthesia. The anaesthetic agent used must provide rapid induction, a fairly deep level of anaesthesia for a few minutes, a rapid return to complete alertness and freedom from post-anaesthetic complications such as vomiting.

"Brietal" has proved very suitable and free from complications; far from finding the induction of anaesthesia unpleasant, most of these patients were astonished or frankly incredulous when told they had been asleep at all. The brief period of retrograde amnesia induced, is a most useful aspect of the drug.

Illustration of the use of continuous methohexitone will now be described in general, neuro- and vascular surgery. The 0.1 % solution is the concentration of my choice and although some other anaesthetists (e.g. R. A. GREEN) suggest higher concentrations they also use a higher total dosage – but the total dose should average 100–300 mg per hour – even though it is quite safe to give up to 5 g in all over a period of 5 hrs.

For pelvic surgery of, for example, the rectum, bladder, prostate and uterus, regional analgesia is provided by an extra-dural block, while the "Brietal" can be used to maintain sleep so that the procedure is made aesthetic for both patient and operator. Similary, in cervical vascular surgery, regional analgesia is obtained with appropriate paraventrical blockade and the patient roused for assessment of neurological sequelae when the common or internal carotid arteries are clamped.

"Brietal" infusion has proved ideal as an anaesthetic agent in the management of patients during stereotactic surgery; for the treatment of Parkinsonism; abnormal movements; intractable pain, implant of gold seeds and rarely for epilepsy. The majority of these patients are elderly and hypertensive, postencephalitic and arteriosclerotic. They react poorly to stress situations, become unaccountably hypothermic and frequently present chest problems. Speech disturbance, slow mentation and emotional lability and apprehension often complicate the depressing picture.

Using the LEKSELL apparatus the patient is placed in a sitting position while he is awake and co-operative. Analgesia, or lack of awareness, is required for fixing the frame on the skull and for the subsequent air-encephalogram. While x-rays are taken and developed in the sitting and supine position the patient can be fully awake. Sleep is induced again while the burr hole is made but during the period that follows   of stimulation and assessment for making the lesion and while the results are being accurately assessed

– it is essential for the patient to be fully conscious and co-operative. Galla-mine triethiodide is used in small doses to reduce muscular power in those patients where abnormal movements are severe and who would otherwise require a larger dose of methohexitone. In this type of administration it is essential that the same team of surgeons and anaesthetists establish an early rapport with the patient; gain his confidence; invite his co-operation and perform the actual operation.

Mention of these methods has been given in brief detail to stress that the successful use of "Brietal" by continuous administration will not be achieved by simply "running it in" but requires understanding of the technique employed and problems likely to be encountered.

Methohexitone is a barbiturate and as such a good hypnotic but a poor analgesic. Nevertheless because anaesthesia can be deepened and lightened rapidly "Brietal" can be used to cover short bursts of painful stimuli – but once again this manoeuvre requires practice and careful timing.

Summary

It is hoped that the facts and findings set out in this paper will not only promote discussion but will help to confirm and justify the increasingly high position which "Brietal" is finding in anaesthetics as a general induction and maintenance agent.

Zusammenfassung

Zusammenfassend sei die Hoffnung ausgesprochen, daß die in dieser Arbeit vorgetragenen Fakten und Befunde nicht nur die Diskussion anregen, sondern auch dazu beitragen mögen, die zunehmend hohe Stellung zu be-stätigen und zu rechtfertigen, die Brevimytal unter den Anaesthetika als allgemeines Einleitungs- und Erhaltungsmittel einnimmt.

Methohexital und Neurolept-Analgesie

Von **Ch. Fink** und **Ch. Meier**

Aus der Anaesthesie-Abteilung (Chefarzt: Dr. Ch. Lehmann)
der Chirurg. Klinik und Poliklinik (Direktor: Prof. Dr. G. Maurer)
am Klinikum rechts der Isar der Technischen Universität München

Die Neurolept-Analgesie wird an unserer Abteilung seit 1963 als Routinenarkose durchgeführt. Die Anwendung – besonders beim Risikopatienten – läßt sich aus ihren Vorteilen ableiten. Diese sind:

1. große therapeutische Breite,
2. geringe Toxizität bei minimaler Belastung des Stoffwechsels,
3. die Gewährleistung stabiler Herz-Kreislauf-Verhältnisse,
4. ein wirksamer Antischockeffekt,
5. schnelles Wiedererwachen bei erhaltener psychischer Indifferenz und relativer Schmerzfreiheit und
6. seltenes postoperatives Erbrechen.

Durch selektive Beeinflussung von Schlaf, Analgesie, Reflexdämpfung und Muskelerschlaffung unterscheidet sich die Neurolept-Analgesie von den konventionellen Kombinationsnarkosen. Demnach gibt es fließende Übergänge zwischen der reinen Neurolept-Analgesie (Henschel), der kombinierten Neurolept-Analgesie mit dem Zusatz von Barbiturat (De Castro, Mundeleer) bzw. Halothane (Stoffregen) und der herkömmlichen Barbiturat-N_2O-Halothan-Narkose.

Während wir früher ausschließlich die reine Neurolept-Analgesie durchführten, sind wir heute der Ansicht, daß in Fällen, in denen kein ausgesprochenes Risiko besteht, der Zusatz geringfügiger Mengen eines Narkosemittels also nicht als unzumutbare Belastung gewertet werden kann, die Kombination mit einem Hypnotikum schneller zu dem erwünschten Gleichgewicht von Schlaf und Analgesie führt und deshalb bevorzugt werden sollte.

Während andere Autoren den Zusatz von Halothan befürworten, wählen wir kleine Barbituratdosen, weil die negativen Eigenschaften des Halothan, also Verminderung der Herzleistung, Rhythmusstörungen und Leberschädigung im Widerspruch zu den Indikationen der Neurolept-Analgesie stehen.

Wir verwenden weder Propanidid noch Thiopental, um Histaminfreisetzung, eine stärker ausgeprägte Hypotonie in der Einleitungsphase und längeren Nachschlaf zu umgehen, sondern bevorzugen Methohexital, das sich mit dieser Narkoseform hervorragend kombinieren läßt.

Nach einer Dehydrobenzperidol-Gabe von 10–15 mg und einer Fentanyl-Gabe von 0,4–0,5 mg injizieren wir 20–30 mg Methohexital, beatmen einige Sekunden lang mit Sauerstoff und intubieren mit Succinylbischolin. Damit bewirken wir ein störungsfreies Einschlafen, ersparen dem Kranken unangenehme Erinnerungen an den Intubationsvorgang, verkürzen die Einleitungsphase und erzielen schnell einsetzende chirurgische Narkosetiefe.

Die kurze, nach Einleitung der Neurolept-Analgesie eintretende Blutdruck-Senkung wird durch diese geringe Barbituratmenge nicht verstärkt. Eine durch das Barbiturat potenzierte Apnoe nach Fentanyl ist ohne praktische Bedeutung, da die Neurolept-Analgesie an unserer Abteilung grundsätzlich in Intubation durchgeführt wird.

In den Fällen, in denen auch hohe Fentanylgaben keine ausreichende Narkosetiefe bewirken, also bei jungen, kräftigen Patienten, bei Alkoholikern oder Morphinisten, erreichen wir durch fraktionierte Nachinjektionen von 10–30 mg Methohexital eine gute Potenzierung der Narkose. Akustische Wahrnehmungen, über die bei der Handhabung reiner Neurolept-Analgesie wiederholt berichtet wurde, werden dadurch mit Sicherheit ausgeschlossen.

Auch in Situationen, bei denen vorübergehend ein reines Sauerstoff-Angebot erwünscht ist, läßt sich der Zeitraum mit dem Barbiturat überbrücken, ohne daß längerer Nachschlaf befürchtet werden muß.

Bei Hirntumoren ist die Einsparung des Neuroleptikums vorteilhaft, da die extra-pyramidal-motorischen Symptome, wie Rigor, Tremor und motorische Unruhe vermieden werden.

Tabelle 1. *Neuroleptanalgesien mit Brietal*

Fachgebiet	1966	1967	1968	1969	1970 1.1.–30.11.	insgesamt
Chirurgie	214	984	850	800	427	3239
Thoraxchirurgie	106	476	425	300	331	1638
Neurochirurgie	326	249	111	107	121	914
Urologie	127	270	136	113	76	722
Gynäkologie	85	101	73	43	57	359
Oto-Laryngologie	54	55	79	80	153	421
Insgesamt	912	2099	1674	1443	1165	7293

Zur erneuten Narkosevertiefung in der Ausleitungsphase ist das Methohexital dem Fentanyl vorzuziehen, da durch den rascheren Abbau des Kurznarkotikums ein Antidot überflüssig wird. Damit erhalten wir uns den auch nach Beendigung der Narkose anhaltenden analgetischen Effekt des Fentanyl und umgehen dessen atemdepressorische Wirkung.

Ein Antidot sollte nur dann gegeben werden, wenn bei ausreichender Decurarisierung eine Ateminsuffizienz weiterbesteht, wenn ohnehin eine kardio-pulmonale Beeinträchtigung vorliegt oder wenn eine postoperative Überwachung nicht gewährleistet werden kann.

In den Jahren von 1966–1970 kombinierten wir 7293 Neurolept-Analgesien mit Methohexital (Tab. 1). Durch

die kreislaufschonende Wirkung (GOLDMANN),
den vagolytischen und bronchodilatatorischen Effekt,
die geringe Kumulation und
durch kaum vorhandene Beeinflussung der Leberfunktion (BITTRICH)

wurde das Präparat auch in Kombination mit der Neurolept-Analgesie den Anforderungen an eine Narkose bei größeren Eingriffen gerecht.

Zusammenfassung

Es werden Anwendungsmöglichkeiten und Vorteile der Kombination einer Neuroleptanalgesie mit Methohexital dargestellt. Sie hat in den Fällen Berechtigung, in denen kein ausgesprochenes Risiko besteht. Methohexital kann hier sowohl bei der Einleitung und der Unterhaltung als auch bei der Ausleitung der Narkose gegeben werden. Die Kombination bürgt für ein störungsfreies und schnelles Einschlafen, schließt Rückerinnerungen und akustische Wahrnehmungen aus, ermöglicht ein zeitweises höheres Sauerstoffangebot und kann die letzte Fentanylgabe ersetzen, die unter Umständen ein Antidot erfordert, das den analgetischen Effekt des Präparates aufhebt.

Summary

The range of application, as well as the advantages of the combination of neuroleptanalgesia with administration of methohexital is demonstrated. It is justified in cases which constitute no pronounced risk. Here methohexital may be used both for induction and maintenance of anaesthesia, as well as in its terminal phase. This combination ensures undisturbed and rapid onset of sleep, excluding memory and acoustic perceptions. It permits the oxygen supply to be transiently increased, and it is able to replace the final administration of Fentanyl which, under certain circumstances, may require application of an antidote which, in turn, might counteract the analgesic effect of the drug.

Literatur

1. Bauer-Ehnes, H. Hölzinger, J.: Zunehmende Anwendung des Methohexital. III. Europ. Anästhesiekongress, Prag 1970.
2. Brand, L.: Physiologic disposition of Methohexital in man. Anesthesiology 24, 331 (1963).
3. Bergmann, H.: Zur NLA mit Phenoperidin und Haloperidol. Anaesthesist 11, 109 (1962).
4. — Indikationen und Kontraindikationen zur NLA. Wien. Med. Wschr. 117, 673 (1967).
5. Bellville, J. W., Fennel, P. J., Marphy, T., Howland, W. S.: The relative potencies of Methohexital and Thiopental. J. Pharmacol. Exp. Ther. 129, 108 (1960).
6. Bittrich, M. M., Kane, A. V. R., Mosher, R. E.: Methohexital and its effect on liver function tests. Anesthesiology 24, 81 (1963).
7. de Castro, J., Mundeleer, P.: Die NLA, Auswahl der Präparate, Bedeutung der Analgesie und der Neurolepsie. Anaesthesist 11, 10 (1962).
8. Colemann, J., Green, R. A.: Methohexital, a short acting barbiturate Anaesthesia 15, 411 (1960).
9. Corssen, G.: Neuroleptanalgesia and anaesthesia. Anesthesia, Analgesie 43, 748 (1964).
10. DelaHaye-Plouvier, G., Cathelin, M., Gaveau, T., Viars, P.: Possibilités et Limites de l'emploi du Fentanyl associé au Droperidol chez des Malades en Respiration Spontanée Anest., Anal., Réan. 27, 682 (1970).
11. Dundee, J. W.: Clinical studies of induction agents. A comparison of eight intravenous anaesthetics as main agents for a standart operation. Brit. J. Anaesth. 35, 784 (1961).
12. — Riding, J. E., Barron, D. W., Nicoll, R. M.: Some factors influencing the introduction characteristics of Methohexital anaesthesia. Brit. J. Anaesth. 33, 296 (1962).
13. Eichler, J., Kukulinus, K.: Epontolnarkose zur Einleitung der NLA. Prakt. Anästh. Wiederbeleb. 18, 207 (1966).
14. Frey, R., Kolb, E.: Fortschritte der Anaesthesiologie. Dtsch. Med. Wschr. 89, 1677 (1964).
15. Grabow, L., Allemand, H. L.: Die Anwendung der NLA in der Herzchirurgie. Anästh. Wiederbeleb. 18, 72 (1966).
16. Goldmann, V., Harris, P.: Intravenous induction of anaesthesia in the dental chair. Brit. Dent. J. 114, 62 (1963).
17. Henschel, W. F.: NLA-Klinik und Fortschritte. III. Bremer NLA-Symposium, Bremen, 21.–22. 5. 1966. Stuttgart: F. K. Schattauer 1967.
18. — Peters, W.: Intravenöse Narkose. Zschr. prakt. Anästh. Wiederbeleb. 6, 417 (1968).
19. Kampferer, J. M.: Prinzipielle und praktische Überlegungen zur NLA. Anaesth. 11, 25 (1962).
20. Lehmann, Ch., Elgert, K., Weber, K.: Erfahrungen mit 5000 Methohexital-Kurznarkosen. Zschr. F. Prakt. Anaesth. Wiederbeleb. 6, 387 (1966).
21. Sabathié, M.. Drei Jahre Verwendung von Dextromoramid in der Anaesthesiologie. Anaesth. 11, 20 (1962).

22. Schellenberger, A., Doenicke, A., Gürtner, Th.: Klinische und tierexperimentelle Untersuchungen zur Leberbelastung nach NLA. Z. f. Anaesth. Wiederbelebung **18**, 8 (1966).
23. Schmidt, K.: Zur Kreislaufwirkung der kombinierten NLA. Z. f. Anaesth. Wiederbelebung **18**, 99 (1966).
24. Stoffregen, J., Schorer, R.: Neuroleptanalgesie und Kombinationsnarkose Z. f. Anaesth. Wiederbelebung **18**, 95 (1966).
25. Taylor, C., Stoelting, V. K.: Methohexital sodium – a new ultrashort acting barbiturate. Anaesth. **21**, 29 (1960).
26. Wyant, G. M., Zoerb, D. L.: Propanidid – a new nonbarbiturate intravenous anaesthetic. Canad. Anaesth. Soc. J. **12**, 569 (1965).

Vergleichende Untersuchungen der kurzwirkenden Barbiturate

Von **R. Frey**

Aus dem Institut für Anaesthesiologie der Universitätskliniken Mainz
(Direktor: Prof. Dr. R. FREY)

Die intravenöse Anaesthesie gilt heute als die verbreitetste Anaesthesiemethode der Welt. Sie hat jedoch nicht nur Vorteile (sie ist todleicht), sondern auch Nachteile (der Patient ist leicht tot). Die Barbiturate führen primär schon zu einer zentralen Atemdepression im Gegensatz zu der Äthernarkose, die ja zunächst die Atmung anregt (Abb. 1).

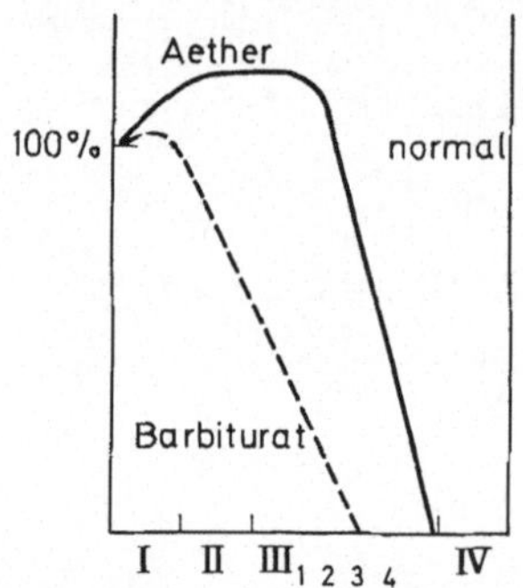

Abb. 1. Die Wirkung der Barbiturate und des Äthers auf die Atmung (schematisch)

Als *Indikationen* gelten:

1. Kurze Eingriffe ohne Erschlaffung (aber auch hier: O_2!).
2. Einleitung und Basis längerer Anaesthesien (häufig Barbiturat, N_2O, Relaxans. Vorteil: Keine Explosionsgefahr).
3. Amnesie bei Lokal- oder Spinalanaesthesie.
4. Antidot von Krampfgiften aus der Lokalanaesthesiereihe.

Als relative *Kontraindikationen* der reinen Barbituratnarkose gelten:

1. Extreme Jugend und Alter.

2. Empfindlichkeit gegen Sauerstoffmangel: Organschaden (Myokard, Leber, Nieren, Atmungsorgane),
Anämie und Schock,
Vergiftung (Coma, Azidose),
Geburtshilfe (Atemdepression des Neugeborenen).

3. Eingriffe in reflexogenen Zonen: Kopf, Hals, alle größeren Eingriffe.

Absolute Kontraindikationen werden heute kaum mehr anerkannt, denn wir haben ja die Gefahren, die drohen (Atemstillstand, Blutdruckabfall usw.), sehr viel besser in der Hand als früher.

Behandlung der *Überdosierung* von Barbituraten:

1. Sauerstoffgabe.
2. Freihaltung der Atemwege.
3. Künstliche Beatmung.
4. Keine Analeptika, da Steigerung des Sauerstoffbedarfs (Krampfgifte).

Vorsichtsmaßregeln: Bei der Barbituratnarkose sollten immer bereitstehen:

1. Ein Beatmungsgerät (ein Atembeutel oder ein Narkoseapparat mit Sauerstoff).
2. Endotrachealtuben und Rachentuben, Laryngoskop und Relaxantien.
3. Verdünnung der Lösung auf 1 % (Methohexital) oder zumindest 2,5 % (alle übrigen Barbiturate).

Es hat sich gezeigt, daß alle Kreislaufwirkungen der Barbiturate und Thiobarbiturate sehr viel geringer sind, wenn gleichzeitig Sauerstoff oder zumindest ein hochprozentiges Sauerstoffgemisch geatmet wird.

Und zum Schluß die *Vorteile* und Nachteile nochmals gegenüber gestellt: Die Einleitung ist angenehm und rasch, Erbrechen ist selten, keine Schleimhautreizung, keine vermehrte Speichelsekretion und die Homöostase wird bei korrekter Durchführung und Sauerstoffgabe kaum beeinträchtigt

Demgegenüber steht doch eine Reihe von *Nachteilen*: Die Analgesie ist bei alleiniger Barbituratnarkose schlecht, wir geben deshalb gerne Lachgas dazu. Die Rachenreflexe sind erhalten; wenn wir also intubieren wollen, müssen wir relaxieren: die Muskelerschlaffung ist unbefriedigend, die Atemdepression ist regelmäßig, und Excitation, Husten und Glottiskrampf sind verhältnismäßig häufig. Die Steuerbarkeit ist gering, besonders bei den länger wirkenden Mitteln, sie wird immer besser, je kürzer die Wirkung dauert. Bei Methohexital kann man schon von einer relativen Steuerbarkeit sprechen.

Wir haben die *dosis hypnotica* verschiedener Barbiturate im Selbstversuch getestet und haben folgende Dosen festgestellt: bei Baytinal etwa 8 mg/kg, bei Cito-Eunarcon etwa 7 mg/kg, bei Thiogenal etwa 6 mg/kg, bei Thiopental etwa 3–4 mg/kg und – Sie haben es heute früh gehört – bei Methohexital ist es 1 mg/kg, also eine wesentlich stärkere Wirkung.

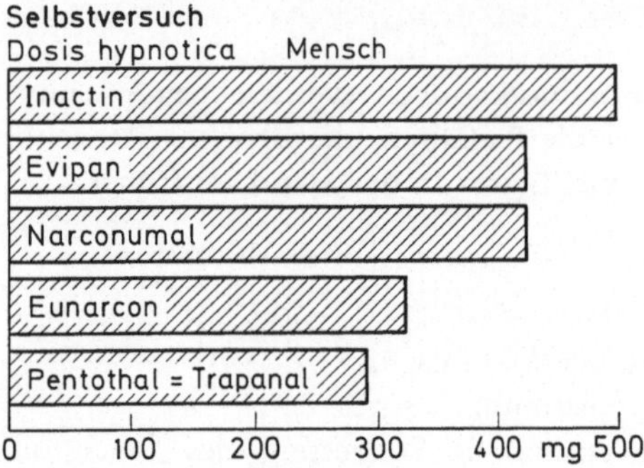

Abb. 2. Die Dosis hypnotica des Methohexital beträgt beim 70 kg schweren Menschen ca. 70 mg. Die Einschlafdosen der anderen Barbiturate sind in der Abbildung wiedergegeben (Selbstversuch von NANKE)

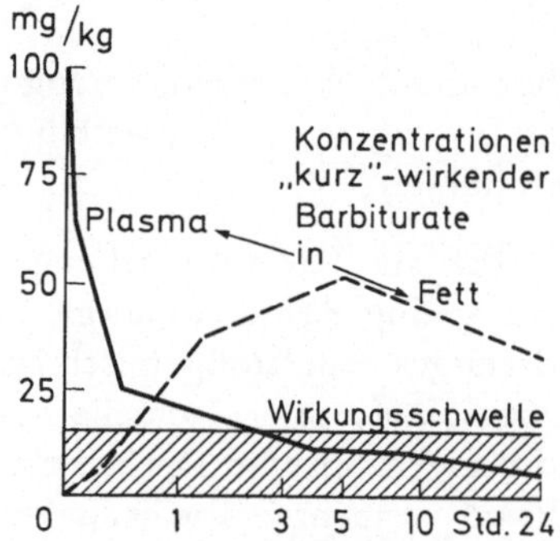

Abb. 3. Konzentration „kurz" wirkender Thio-Barbiturate im Plasma und im Fett (schematisch)

Nun die *Gesamtdosen,* die für das Einschlafen benötigt wurden. Sie betrugen beim Inactin 500 mg, beim Evipan 400 mg, beim Narconumal 350–400 mg, beim Eunarkon etwa 300 mg und beim Thiopental etwa 200–300 mg. Beim Methohexital waren es – entsprechend der Kilogrammzahl der Versuchspersonen – 50–70 mg.

Nun die *Verteilung im Plasma:* Im Plasma sinkt der Spiegel dieser Barbiturate binnen Minuten rasch ab und erreicht unterschwellige Werte; deshalb eben das schnelle Erwachen. Während besonders die Thio-Barbiturate sehr viel in das Fett abwandern (Abb. 3), haben wir beim Methohexital diese erhöhte Fettlöslichkeit nicht in dem Maße.

Die *chronischen Vergiftungen:* Bei unseren Rattenversuchen sehen Sie, daß bei ständig erhöhter Dosis[1] schließlich die Tiere nach 35–55 Tagen zugrunde gehen, und zwar bei den Thiobarbituraten schneller als bei den gewöhnlichen Barbituraten (Abb. 4).

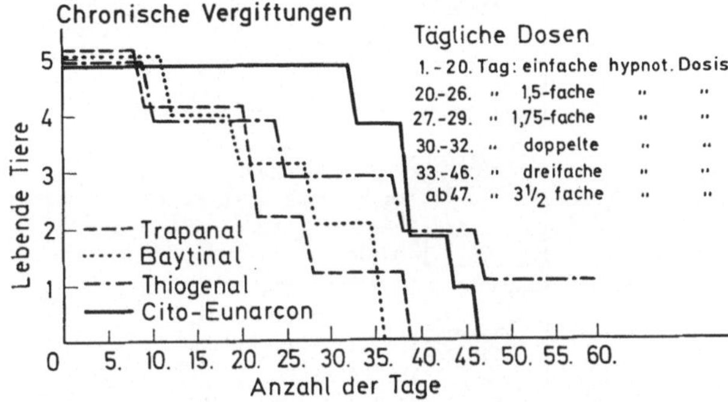

Abb. 4. Chronische Vergiftungen mit Barbituraten und Thiobarbituraten (Ratten-Versuche, NANKE)

Zum Schluß der *Vergleich der Wirkungsdauer* dieser verschiedenen zuletzt diskutierten Mittel: Beim *Thiopental* 5 mg/kg (die Einschlafdosis, die wir vorhin diskutiert haben); in der Reihenfolge der Säulen ist oben die Einschlafzeit (das ist eine knappe Minute), dann die Toleranzzeit (wieder etwa 2 min) und die Aufwachzeit (wieder 1–2 min) angegeben. Unten der lange schwarze Balken bedeutet die Erholungszeit: so lange braucht der Patient, bis seine Reflexe alle wieder da sind, bis er wieder normal auf Zuruf reagiert, bis auch die psychomotorischen Reflexe wieder in Ordnung sind (diese Versuche wurden in Mainz von Herrn KREUSCHER durchgeführt). Dann beim *Epontol:* die Einschlafzeit und die Aufwachzeit sind etwas verkürzt (die Toleranzzeit sogar etwas länger); aber die *Erholungszeit,* bis alle Reflexe wieder normal sind, ist wesentlich kürzer: oben 80 min (Thiopental) und unten dann etwa 10–20 min (Propanidid). Ganz ähnlich sind diese Zeiten beim Methohexital: Auch da relativ ordentliche Toleranzzeit, sehr kurze Aufwachzeit und genauso kurze Erholungszeit bis zur Rückkehr aller Reflexe, wie beim Propanidid (Epontol) (Abb. 5).

---

[1] 1.–20. Tag: Einfache Dosis hypnotica; 20.–26. Tag: 1,5-fache; 27.–29. Tag: 1,75-fache; 30.–32. Tag: Doppelte; 33.–46. Tag: Dreifache; ab 47. Tag: 3,5-fache Dosis hypnotica.

   Nun sind folgende *Fragen* noch zu beantworten (vielleicht helfen hierbei die Experten aus dem Auditorium): Wir haben heute früh bei der Pharmakologie in einer Kurve gesehen, daß der Spiegel des Methohexital im
Blut doch relativ langsam abfällt; das zieht sich doch über Stunden hin.

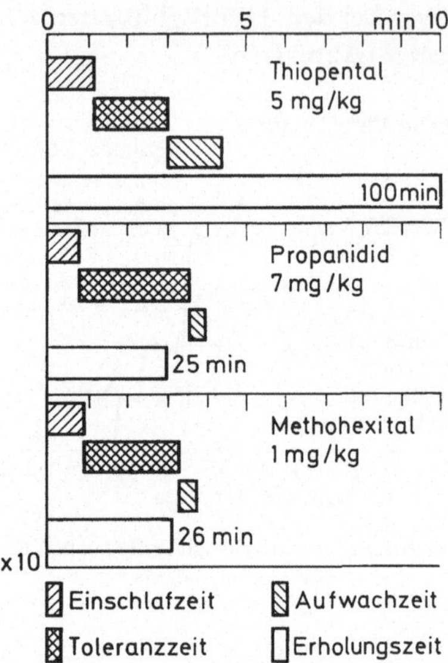

Abb. 5. Einschlafzeit, Toleranzzeit und Aufwachzeit nach Injektion dreier Kurznarkotika beim Menschen. Die Erholungszeit ist mit einer anderen Zeitschreibung
gezeichnet (muß mit 10 multipliziert werden). (Modifiziert nach Kreuscher)

Warum ist dann die Wirkung so kurz und warum sind diese Patienten so
schnell doch ganz wieder da, auch mit allen ihren Reflexen? Anscheinend
ist es so, daß doch ein Teil relativ rasch abgebaut wird und dann ein anderer
Teil verteilt wird in den großen Flüssigkeitsräumen des Körpers, die ja
teilweise schlechter durchblutet sind, so daß dadurch ein relativ rasches Verschwinden aus dem Blut und ein rascher Abfall des Spiegels im Plasma eintritt, der allerdings dann sich asymptotisch ausschleicht, so daß ich die volle
Verkehrstüchtigkeit dieser Patienten nicht anerkennen würde; ich würde
also auch nach Methohexital-Narkose empfehlen, die Patienten nur im Auto,
und zwar nicht im selbst gesteuerten Auto, sondern sitzend in einer Taxe
z.B. nach Hause zu entlassen, unter Begleitung eines verantwortlichen Erwachsenen, nicht auf eigene Verantwortung. Insofern bedeutet eben die
kürzere Wirkungszeit dieses Mittels einen großen Fortschritt: man kann
die Patienten schneller entlassen; aber dies bedeutet nicht, daß man sie allein
fortlassen darf.

Zusammenfassung

Ausgehend von den Vor- und Nachteilen der verschiedenen intravenösen Narkotika werden die Einschlafdosen, die Toleranz- und die Aufwachzeiten dieser Mittel am Menschen verglichen, ebenso die Wirkung chronischer Vergiftungen im Tierversuch. Hierbei zeigte sich, daß Methohexital neben Propanidid das am kürzesten wirkende Mittel ist und stärker wirkt als andere vergleichbare Kurznarkotika.

Die Straßenfähigkeit im „Alleingang" wird jedoch – wie bei allen i. v.-Narkotica – erst am nächsten Tag erreicht. In Begleitung kann der Patient jedoch meist genauso früh nach Hause gehen, wie bei dem einzig vergleichbaren Mittel, dem Eugenolderivat Propanidid, d. h. oft schon nach 1 Std. Dies bedeutet eine wesentliche Entlastung unserer Ambulanzen.

Summary

Starting from the advantages and disadvantages of the various intravenous anaesthetics, the doses required for inducing sleep, the times of tolerance, and the waking-up times of these drugs in the human are compared, as are the effects of chronic toxicity in animal experiments. Here, methohexital is shown to be the drug with the shortest-lasting activity next to propanidide and to produce a more pronounced effect than other short-acting anaesthetics.

Street safety, however, is not regained by the patient until the next day, however, this applies to all intravenous anaesthetics. But when accompanied, the patient may generally go home just as soon as following propanidide anaesthesia (this is a eugenol derivative and is the only comparable drug), that means to say mostly already one hour after awakening. This imples a considerable relief to our ambulances.

Literatur

Frey, R.: Langenbecks Archiv klin. Chir. **282**, 177 (Kongreßband 1955); dort weitere Literatur.
Haas, E., H. Kreuscher und M. Strickstrock: Anaesthesist **12**, 346 (1963).
Nanke, E.: Diss. med. Heidelberg 1955.

Untersuchungen hinsichtlich der Straßenfähigkeit nach Methohexital- und Propanidid-Narkosen

Von **O. Darboven**

Aus der Anaesthesie-Abteilung (Chefarzt: Dr. CH. LEHMANN)
der Chirurg. Klinik und Poliklinik (Direktor: Prof. Dr. G. MAURER)
am Klinikum rechts der Isar der Technischen Universität München

Die Vorteile der intravenösen Kurznarkose, also
schnelles, angenehmes Einschlafen,
rasch einsetzende Narkosetiefe mit ausreichender Analgesie
und kurze Erholungsphasen ohne unangenehme Nachwirkungen
sind allgemein bekannt.

Das rasche Abklingen der Narkosewirkung ist eine der wichtigsten
Voraussetzungen für die Eignung eines intravenösen Kurznarkotikums in
der ambulanten Praxis, weil Überwachungspersonal und Liegeräume in
vielen Fällen fehlen. Andererseits verpflichtet der Gesetzgeber den Arzt,
den Patienten erst dann zu entlassen, wenn die Wirkung des Anaesthetikums
abgeklungen ist.

Daher ist es naheliegend, festzustellen, inwieweit Kurznarkotika die
Straßenfähigkeit beeinträchtigen.

Wir stellten uns die Aufgabe, die Wirkung von Methohexital und Propanidid hinsichtlich der Straßenverkehrstauglichkeit zu prüfen.

Um vergleichbare Resultate zu erhalten, führten wir insgesamt 60 Versuche an 30 etwa gleichaltrigen Medizinstudenten durch, denen innerhalb
von 45 sec in der ersten Versuchsreihe 2 mg Methohexital pro kg Körpergewicht und in der zweiten Versuchsreihe, die eine Woche später erfolgte,
5 mg Propanidid pro kg Körpergewicht injiziert wurden.

Weil wir die Überlagerung mehrerer Präparate ausschließen wollten,
verzichteten wir auf jegliche Prämedikation.

Vor der Injektion der Betäubungsmittel und während der Aufwachzeit
wurden Blutdruck, Puls und Atmung fortlaufend kontrolliert. Zusätzlich
registrierten wir Apnoe, Singultus, Husten, Laryngospasmus und Muskelzuckungen.

Als Aufwachzeit maßen wir die Zeit vom Beginn der Injektion bis
zu dem Moment, in dem die Versuchsperson auf Aufforderung die Augen
öffnete.

Eine halbe Stunde vor Narkosebeginn wurden 3 Tests, eine Reaktions-, eine Überblicks- und eine Konzentrations-Prüfung durchgeführt, die wir 30 und 60 min nach der Injektion von Methohexital bzw. Propanidid wiederholten.

Wir wählten solche Reaktionsproben, deren Validität oder Rechtsgültigkeit und Stabilität bekannt sind und die sich allein in München bei über 20000 Fahrtauglichkeitsuntersuchungen bewährten.

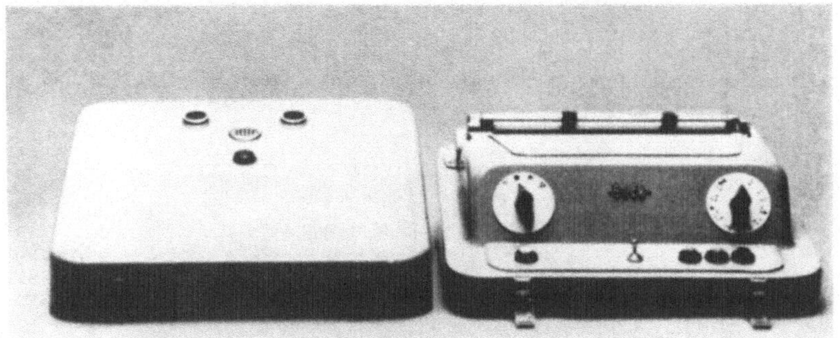

Abb. 1. Reaktionszeitmesser nach Beck

Zunächst wurde die Reaktionszeitmessung am Beck-Gerät durchgeführt, die eine auf $^1/_{100}$ sec genaue Messung der Reaktionszeit sowohl auf optische oder akustische Reize allein, als auch auf deren variierte Konstellationen erlaubt.

Die Bedeutung der isoliert gemessenen Reaktionszeit für ein verkehrssicheres Verhalten wird im allgemeinen weitgehend überschätzt. Gerade unter dem Einfluß von Medikamenten aber sind Reaktionszeitverlängerungen bekannt, die im modernen Straßenverkehr gefährliche Folgen nach sich ziehen können.

Im zweiten Test legt die Versuchsperson eine Arbeitsprobe am Tensor nach Beck ab, deren Ergebnis Rückschlüsse auf die Art der optischen Aufmerksamkeitsverteilung gestattet (Abb. 2).

Dem Probanden wird – wie das Bild erkennen läßt – eine Tafel gezeigt, auf der in ungeordneter und teilweise wiederholter Folge die Ziffern 1 bis 40 verzeichnet sind. Die einzelnen Zahlen wurden jeweils mit einem von 10 verschiedenen Verkehrszeichen gekoppelt, die sich auf einem schreibmaschinenartigen Registriergerät mit 10 Tasten wiederfinden. Die Prüflinge haben die dargebotenen Ziffern durch das Niederdrücken der entsprechenden Taste zu verarbeiten. Eine Schreibvorrichtung erstellt ein Protokollblatt, von dem zu entnehmen ist, welche Zeit die Versuchsperson von Ziffer zu Ziffer benötigte, um die entsprechende Taste mit dem ihr zugehörenden Verkehrszeichen zu finden.

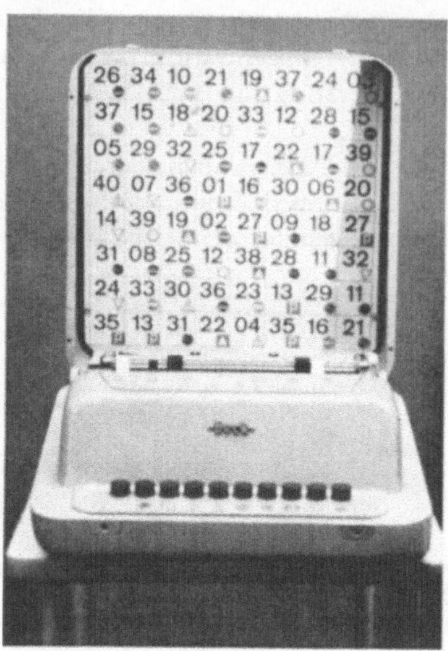

Abb. 2. Tensor nach Beck

Die dritte Aufgabe bestand im sogenannten „Test d2". Die Probe verlangt, 14 Druckzeilen so rasch und so sorgfältig als möglich auf das Vorkommen von 3 bestimmten Zeichen, die durchgestrichen werden müssen, zu überprüfen. Der Proband hat für jede Zeile 20 sec Zeit, ehe er aufgefordert wird, mit der nächsten zu beginnen.

Das Verfahren ermöglicht in erster Linie Feststellungen darüber, ob sich ein Mensch im Bereich der optischen Wahrnehmung während längerer Zeit auf das Bemerken bestimmter Elemente, die unregelmäßig in einer Fülle verschiedener Zeichen verteilt sind, konzentrieren kann. Diese Aufgabe regt durch ihre besondere Struktur zur geistigen Tätigkeit an, bewirkt jedoch so starke Ablenkungen, daß ihre einwandfreie Lösung in Frage gestellt wird. Ähnlich wird auch das Sich-Konzentrieren im Straßenverkehr, also das Bemühen, Vorgänge rational zu erfassen, bewußt zu verarbeiten und sie in unmittelbare Reaktionen umzusetzen, erheblich beeinträchtigt (Abb. 3).

Schließlich wurde festgestellt, nach welchem Zeitraum das physische und psychische Verhalten der Versuchspersonen wieder „normal" war und wann sie ohne Begleitung entlassen werden konnten.

Alle Probanden schliefen innerhalb von 15–20 sec, noch bevor die gesamte Dosis des Narkotikums injiziert worden war, ein.

Vorwiegend nach Methohexital wurden Schmerzen an der Injektionsstelle angegeben.

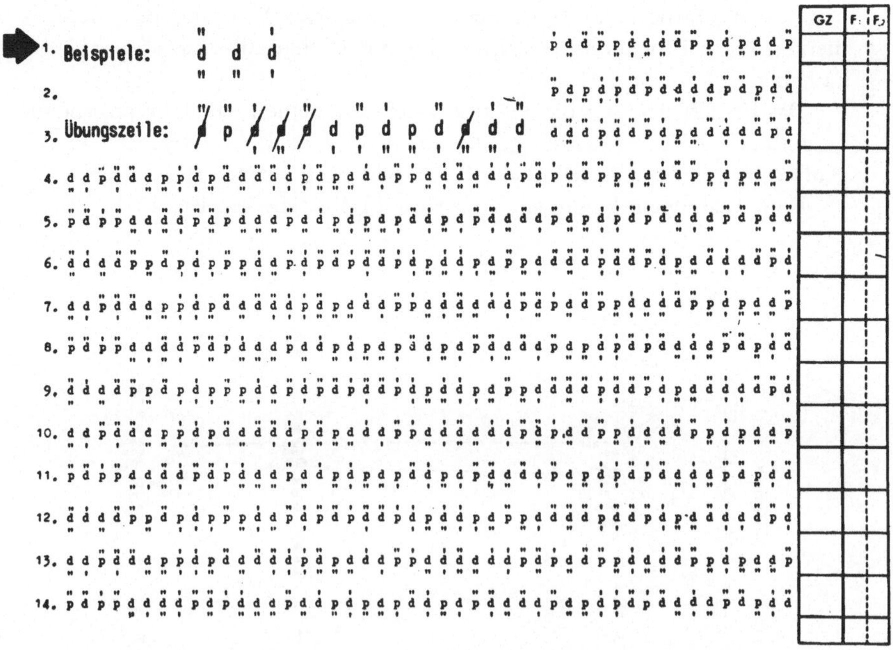

Abb. 3. Test d2

Infolge der langsamen Injektionszeit von 45 sec traten nur vereinzelt kurze apnoische Phasen von höchstens 20 sec Dauer ein.

Im weiteren Verlauf konnten wir hinsichtlich ihrer Wirkung auf die Atmung keine Unterschiede zwischen den Mitteln feststellen.

Beide Anaesthetika bewirkten einen vorübergehenden Abfall des systolischen Blutdruckes. Die Senkung betrug nach Methohexital durchschnittlich 15 mmHg, nach Propanidid im Mittel 30 mmHg. Synchron mit der Abnahme des Blutdruckes nahm die Pulsfrequenz zu. Diese Beobachtungen decken sich mit den von DOENICKE und anderen durchgeführten Untersuchungen.

Während der Methohexital-Narkose traten in 8 Fällen Singultus, in 6 Fällen Zuckungen der Extremitäten und in 2 Fällen unruhige Bewegungen der Arme und Beine, während der Propanidid-Narkose in einem Fall Pulsarrhythmien auf.

Niesen, Laryngospasmus, Emesis und Exantheme wurden weder nach Methohexital noch nach Propanidid beobachtet.

Die Aufwachzeit betrug nach Methohexital durchschnittlich 7 min, nach Propanidid 2–4 min. Alle Versuchspersonen erwachten rasch, waren innerhalb einer Minute zeitlich und örtlich orientiert und gaben sofort

und unaufgefordert Auskunft über die subjektive Wirkung des Medika-
mentes. Nach Propanidid bestritten einige Prüflinge, überhaupt geschlafen
zu haben.

Das Einschlafen und die Träume wurden in beiden Fällen als angenehm
geschildert. Zwei Studenten gaben an, daß sie nach Methohexital in der
Aufwachphase haschischähnliche Halluzinationen hatten.

Eine Testperson klagte nach Propanidid über starken Brechreiz.

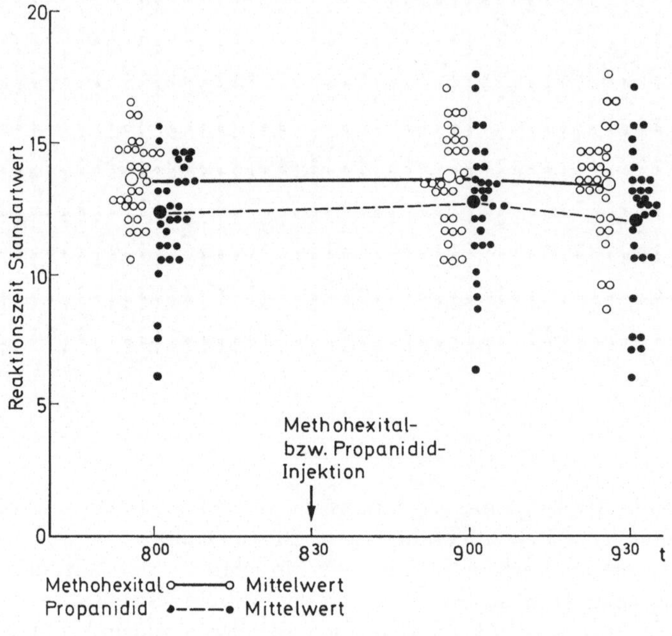

Abb. 4.

Nach beiden Narkosen bestand eine ausgeprägte Fusionsschwäche. Ein
Drittel der gesamten Testpersonen sah Doppelbilder, die bei Propanidid
nach 20 min, bei Methohexital nach 30 min verschwanden.

15 min nach der Methohexital- bzw. Propanidid-Injektion waren alle
Versuchspersonen in der Lage, mit geschlossenen Augen aufrecht und
ohne größere Schwankungen zu stehen.

Die psychodiagnostischen Tests führten zu folgenden Resultaten:

Die durchschnittliche Reaktionszeit auf optische und akustische Reize
betrug vor Narkosebeginn mit Methohexital 13,4, 30 min nach der Injektion
13,5 und 60 min nach der Injektion 13,4 Standardwert. Die Reaktionszeit
blieb also nach Methohexital unverändert.

Auch nach den Propanididnarkosen blieben die Standardwerte der Reaktionszeit annähernd konstant. Sie betrugen 12,9, 12,6 und 12,0 Standardwert. Hier muß der durch die vorher durchgeführte Methohexitalnarkose erworbene Übungsfaktor in Betracht gezogen werden (Abb. 4).

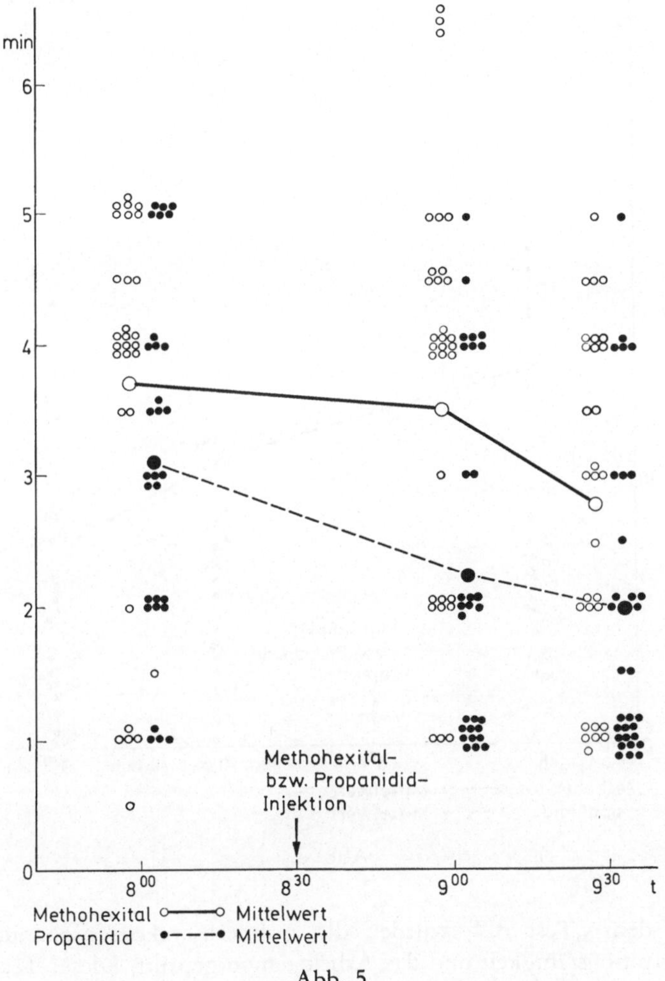

Abb. 5.

Bei der Untersuchung am Beck'schen Tensor nahmen Auffassungsgabe und Konzentrationsfähigkeit in beiden Fällen nach der Narkose zu. Da jedoch der Übungsfaktor auch in diesem Fall eine wesentliche Rolle spielt, wäre lediglich eine Verschlechterung gegenüber dem Ausgangswert ausschlaggebend. Methohexital rangierte hier vor Propanidid (Abb. 5).

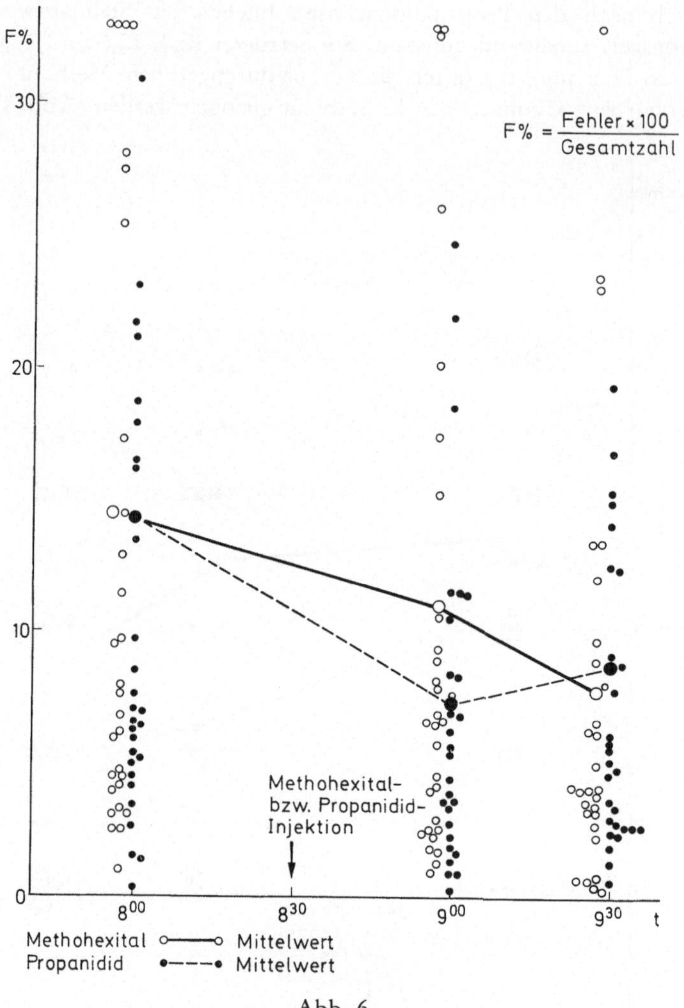

Abb. 6.

Mit dem „Test d2" wurden die Aufmerksamkeitsanspannung, die Konzentrationsfähigkeit und das Arbeitstempo geprüft. Dieser Test zeigte einen unerwarteten Unterschied zwischen der postnarkotischen Phase nach Methohexital und Propanidid. Während die Prozentzahl der Fehler nach Methohexital, das in der ersten Versuchsreihe gegeben wurde, also keine Anpassung für sich in Anspruch nehmen kann, stetig abnahm, war 1 Std nach der Propanididinjektion ein Anstieg der Prozentzahl der Fehler zu verzeichnen. Nach Propanidid trat also ein Nachlassen der Aufmerksamkeitsanspannung und der Konzentrationsfähigkeit auf (Abb. 6).

Als postnarkotische psychische Störungen beobachteten wir bei beiden Präparaten Euphorie, mangelnde Selbstkritik und leichte Enthemmung. Spätestens 90 min nach Methohexital und 60 min nach Propanidid wurde die psychische Ausgangslage jedoch wieder erreicht.

Die Untersuchungen zeigten, daß bezüglich der Narkose-Einleitung, der hypnotischen Wirkung und der postnarkotischen psychischen Veränderungen zwischen Methohexital und Propanidid keine signifikanten Unterschiede bestehen.

Zusammenfassung

Zur Überprüfung der Straßenfähigkeit nach Kurznarkosen mit Methohexital bzw. Propanidid wurden folgende Untersuchungen durchgeführt:

1. Am „Reaktionszeitmesser nach Beck" wurde die Reaktionszeit sowohl auf optische oder akustische Reize allein, als auch auf deren variierte Konstellationen geprüft.

2. Am „Tensor nach Beck" wurde die optische Aufmerksamkeitsverteilung ermittelt.

3. Mit dem Test „d2" wurden Arbeitstempo und Konzentrationsvermögen untersucht.

Die 3 Tests wurden eine halbe Stunde vor Narkosebeginn durchgeführt und 30 und 60 min nach der Injektion von Methohexital bzw. Propanidid wiederholt.

Die Untersuchungsergebnisse zeigten, daß 90 min nach der Methohexital- und 60 min nach der Propanidid-Injektion die psychische Ausgangslage wieder erreicht war.

Bezüglich der Narkose-Einleitung, der hypnotischen Wirkung und der postnarkotischen psychischen Veränderungen bestehen zwischen Methohexital und Propanidid keine signifikanten Unterschiede.

Summary

The following examinations were performed with the aim of assessing the street safety after short anaesthesia with methohexital or propanidide:

1. With the "Beck device" the reaction time both to optic and to acoustic stimuli alone, and to various combinations of these stimuli was examined.

2. Employing the "Tensor according to Beck", the optic attention distribution was registered.

3. Applying the "d2 Test", the working pace and the concentration capacity were studied.

These three tests were carried out one half hour prior to the beginning of anaesthesia and were repeated 30 and 60 minutes, after the injection of methohexital or propanidide injection.

The results obtained in these examinations showed that the original mental condition was recovered 90 minutes after injection of methohexital and 60 minutes after propanidide.

With regard to the induction of anaesthesia, the hypnotic effects and the postanaesthetic mental alterations there exist no significant differences between these two drugs.

Literatur

BINKERT, E.: Vergleichende Untersuchungen über die Straßenverkehrstauglichkeit nach Thiopental und Methohexital-Kurznarkosen. Schweiz. Med. Wschr. **91**, 1285 (1961).

BIRKENKAMP, R.: Test „d 2"-Aufmerksamkeits-Belastungs-Test. Verlag für Psychologie, Dr. C. J. Hogrefe, Göttingen, S. 7–49 (1962).

CLARKE, R. S. J., DUNDEE, J. W.: Vorläufige Beobachtungen mit einem neuen Phenoxyessigsäure-Derivat Propanidid. Vortrag auf der Arbeitstagung der Dtsch. Ges. f. Anaesthesie am 25.–26. 1. (1964).

CLIVE, J.: Erholungszeit nach Narkose mit Methohexital. Brit. J. of Anesthesia, **32**, No. 12 (1960).

DANNEMANN, H., LÜBKE, P.: Komplikationen während Narkosen mit Epontol. Z. prakt. Anaesth. **4**, (1970).

DORSCH, W., v. HEBENSTREIT, B.: Die Wirkung eines Fluphenazin-Dihydrochlorids auf die Fahrtauglichkeit. Editio Cantor K. G. Verlag für Medizin und Naturwissenschaften (1964).

DOENICKE, A., KUGLER, J.: Electrical Brain Funktion During Emergence Time after Methohexital and Propanidid. Acta Anaesth. Scand., Supp. **17**, 99 (1965).

DUNDEE, J. W.: Ultrashort-acting Barbiturates for Out-Patients. Acta Anaesth. Scand., Supp. **17**, 17 (1965).

KOCH, L.: Klinische Erfahrungen mit dem neuen intravenösen Kurznarkotikum Propanidid (Epontol). Med. Welt **17**, 901 (1966).

KREUSCHER, H.: Zur Straßenverkehrstüchtigkeit nach Anwendung von Propanidid. Vortrag auf der Arbeitstagung der Dtsch. Ges. f. Anaesthesie am 25.–26. 1. 1964.

RITTMEYER, P.: Weitere Untersuchungen zur Frage der Straßenverkehrstüchtigkeit nach Propanidid-Narkosen. Vortrag auf der Arbeitstagung der Dtsch. Ges. f. Anaesthesie 25.–26. 1. 1964.

ZINDLER, M.: Intravenöse Kurznarkose für ambulante Patienten. Methohexital und Propanidid. Dtsch. Med. Wschr. **35**, S. 1506 (1965).

Methohexital im klinischen Vergleich
mit anderen intravenösen Kurznarkotica

Von **F. Chladek**

Aus der Anaesthesie-Abteilung am Zentralkrankenhaus Links der Weser in Bremen
(Chefarzt: Dr. F. Böhmert)

Wir haben uns Anfang des Jahres 1970 entschlossen, das zwar lange bekannte, aber in unserer Abteilung bisher nicht angewandte Brevimytal einzusetzen, um uns über seine klinischen Eigenschaften ein eigenes Bild zu verschaffen. Unsere Absicht war es, festzustellen, ob unsere Forderungen an ein Kurznarkotikum, nämlich geringstmöglicher Aufwand, schnelle An- und Abflutung, keine Nebenwirkungen, geringe Toxizität und kurzfristiges Wiedereintreten von Kritik- und Reaktionsvermögen, auch von Brevimytal erfüllt werden und ob vor allem im Vergleich mit Thiopental und Propanidid beim Brevimytal wirkliche Vorteile zu registrieren sind.

Schon nach kurzer klinischer Anwendung von Methohexital erschienen uns einige Vorteile dieser Substanz so auffällig, daß wir sie einer systematischen klinischen Studie nach einem speziellen Untersuchungsschema im Vergleich mit Thiopental und Propanidid bei je 50 Patienten unterzogen (Abb. 1).

Eine Großzahl chirurgischer Eingriffe machen nach Ursache und Art der Behandlung ein Verbleiben des Patienten in der Klinik nicht erforderlich. Solche Eingriffe wurden früher meist in Leitungs- oder Lokalanaesthesie durchgeführt. Die an die „Schlafspritze" gewöhnten Patienten wollen aber heute von der chirurgischen Prozedur nichts mehr hören und sehen.

Um einen längeren Krankenhausaufenthalt zu vermeiden, begann man Anfang der fünfziger Jahre sogenannte Ultrakurznarkotika herzustellen und diese klinisch zu erproben. In Amerika war es besonders Methohexital (über klinische Erfahrungen haben zum ersten Mal Gruber und Stoelting im Jahre 1957 berichtet), in Europa standen Eugenolderivate als i. v. Ultrakurznarkotika im Vordergrund.

Die Chemie und Pharmakologie von Methohexital dürfen wir als bekannt voraussetzen. Aufgrund unserer pharmakologischen Kenntnisse über Kurznarkotica hinsichtlich Wirkungseintritt, Dauer und Erholungsphase haben wir für ihre Anwendung eine reiche Indikationsskala (Abb. 2), in der unsere 150 Patienten vergleichend zwischen Methohexital, Thiopental

Name: Sch. Karl		Alter: 43 J.	Datum: 21.9.70	Nr. 64
Ambulant: −	Geschlecht: ♂	Dg.: Bauchdeckenabszeß		
Stationär: +	Gewicht: 78 kg	Op.: Inzision, Drain		
Anaesth. Anamnese u. Befund:		Frühere Narkosen ohne Zwischenfälle. Bereits vor 2 Wochen eine Kurznarkose mit Brevimytal durchgeführt.		
Präoper. Therapie: Antibiotika (Binotal, Stapenor)	Anaesth. Risiko: I	Prämedikation: Atropin: 0,0005 g Thalamonal: 1,5 ml		

Kurznarkotikum: Brevimytal	Zeit	14.40	14.42	14.45	14.49	15.00	15.15
	RR	130/80	120/80	125/80	125/80	130/80	130/80
	Puls	80	76	80	80	76	76
	Atmung	16	12	16	20	16	16
	AMV						
	EKG						
	Blutgase	+	+			+	

	Zeit:	Menge:	Geschw.:
Initialdosis	14.40	100 mg	10 sec
Nachinjektion	14.44	50 mg	10 sec
Gesamtdosis:		150 mg	

Nebenwirkungen und postnark. Störungen:					
Apnoe: ∅					
Atemdepression: Hypoventilation etwa 30 sec nach der Initialdosis					
Arrhythmie: ∅					
Allerg. Reaktion: ∅					
RR-Abfall	±	Muskelzittern u. Tremor	+	Schwindelgefühl	±
Pulsänderung	±	Krämpfe	−	Benommenheit	−
Singultus	−	Brechreiz	−	Venenschmerz	−
Husten, Niesen	−	Erbrechen	−	Defäkation	−
Euphorie	−	Depress. Zustände	−	Kopfschmerzen	−
Anderes:					
Einschlafzeit: 12 sec		Aufwachzeit: 22 sec		Narkosedauer: 9 min	
Erholungszeit: 10 min		Entlassungszeit: Stationär			
Bemerkung: −					

Abb. 1. Untersuchungsprotokoll

und Propanidid enthalten sind. Eine Auswahl des Patientengutes nach Alter, Allgemeinzustand und Anaesthesierisiko wurde im eigentlichen nicht vorgenommen. Der jüngste Patient, der eine i.v. Kurznarkose erhielt, war 5 Jahre, der älteste 92 Jahre alt.

1.	Probeexzisionen	10
2.	Inzisionen	45
3.	Entfernung von Finger- und Zehennägeln	12
4.	Reposition von Luxat. und Frakturen	32
5.	Anlegen und Entfernung von Drahtextensionen	4
6.	Gelenkpunktionen	5
7.	Gelenkbewegung bei Teilversteifungen	3
8.	Schmerzhafter Verbandwechsel	6
9.	Sphinkterdehnung	2
10.	Gynäkologische Kurzeingriffe	19
11.	Zahnextraktionen	12
	Gesamtzahl	150

Abb. 2. Indikationen für Narkose der 150 untersuchten Patienten

Technik: Nach einhalbstündiger vorheriger i.m. Atropin- und Thalamonalgabe bei stationären Patienten oder nach fünfminütiger vorheriger i.v. Atropingabe bei ambulanten erhielten die Patienten i.v. Brevimytal in einer Dosierung von 1–1,5 mg pro Kilogramm des Körpergewichtes in 1%-iger Lösung in 10–15 sec injiziert. Bei Eingriffen, die länger als 3–5 min andauerten und eine Re-Injektion erforderlich machten, haben wir etwa die Hälfte der Initialdosis nachinjiziert und die Narkose hinsichtlich Vertiefung der Analgesie mit Lachgas-Sauerstoff im Verhältnis 3:1 verlängert.

In gleicher Weise haben wir Epontol beim Erwachsenen mit 7–10 mg pro kg Körpergewicht, das sind in der Regel 10 ml der 5%igen Lösung, bzw. Thiopental zwischen 300–500 mg zur Kurznarkose verabfolgt.

Zur Überprüfung der drei Substanzen hinsichtlich ihrer Wirkung auf Atmung und Kreislauf haben wir bei den 50 Patienten jeder Gruppe Kreislaufkontrollen am Monitor Hellige (Blutdruck, Puls, EKG) sowie eine Atemminutenvolumenmessung mit dem Dräger-Volumeter vom Beginn der Narkose über die Aufwachzeit hinaus bis zur Entlassung aus der anaesthesiologischen Betreuung durchgeführt. Mehrere Nachinjektionen eines Kurznarkotikums waren bei unseren Patienten selten notwendig. Sie wurden möglichst vermieden, da eine solche Dauernarkose u. E. dem Wesen und der Anwendung von Ultrakurznarkotica widerspricht.

Unsere Ergebnisse

Narkoseeinleitung: Nach i.v. Injektion von Brevimytal schliefen die Patienten ebenso schnell und ohne Zeichen der Exzitation ein wie beim Epontol, während beim Thiopental die Einschlafzeit deutlich verlängert war (Abb. 3).

		Brevimytal	Thiopental	Epontol
1.	Apnoe	3	3	2
2.	Atemdepression	3	2	2
3.	RR-Abfall	4	2	3
4.	Pulsänderung	(↓)	↓	↑
5.	Allergische Reaktion	4	4	(2)
6.	Singultus, Niesen, Husten	3	3	3
7.	Brechreiz, Erbrechen	3	3	3
8.	Muskelzittern und Tremor	3	4	4
9.	Schwindelgefühl und Benommenheit	4	2	4
10.	Psychische Veränderungen	3	3	4
11.	Einschlafzeit	4	3	4
12.	Exzitation	4	4	4
13.	Aufwachzeit	4	2	4
14.	Erholungsphase	4	1	4

Abb. 3. Ergebnisse. 4 = ausgezeichnet, 3 = gut, 2 = mäßig, 1 = unbefriedigend

Narkoseverlauf: Die Narkosedauer bei unseren Patienten betrug im Mittel 2 bis maximal 10 min. Eine gelegentliche Nachinjektion war bei Brevimytal und Epontol früher notwendig als beim Thiopental, entsprechend dem schnelleren Abbau der beiden ersten Substanzen. Die von vielen Autoren beschriebene Apnoe nach der Einleitung mit Brevimytal haben wir bei unserer Technik in 20% der Fälle beobachtet. Sie betrug im Durchschnitt nicht mehr als 15 sec. Hierin unterschied sich Brevimytal gegenüber Thiopental (bei 25% der Fälle Apnoe von 20 sec) nach unseren Erfahrungen nicht wesentlich.

Beim Epontol haben wir dagegen nach anfänglicher Hyperventilation der Patienten eine Apnoe von 30–50 sec registrieren können.

Blutgasanalytische Untersuchungen vor, während und unmittelbar nach einer Brevimytalnarkose zeigten keine signifikanten Veränderungen (Abb 4).

Die Blutdruckwerte vor und nach der Kurznarkose waren beim Brevimytal und Epontol bei 80% der Fälle unverändert, bei Thiopental mußten wir dagegen am Ende der Narkose immer einen systolischen Blutdruckabfall von 10–30 mmHg registrieren (Abb. 5). Während der Narkose

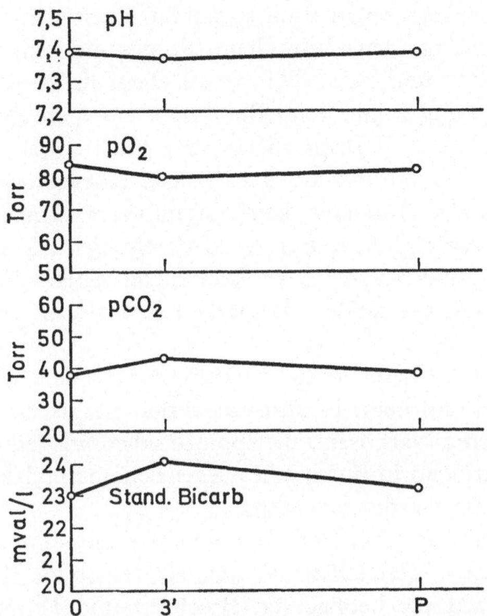

Abb. 4. Blutgasanalysen bei Brevimytal-Kurznarkosen (Durchschnittswerte von 10 Patienten). o = Ausgangswert, 3′ = 3 min nach der Initialdosis, P = 10 min nach dem Erwachen

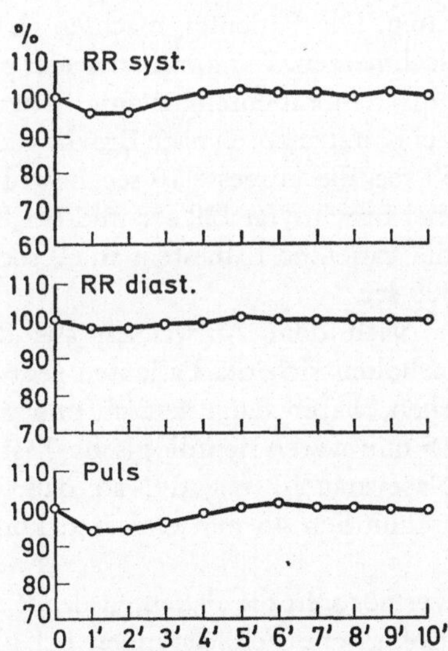

Abb. 5. Mittlere prozentuale Veränderungen von syst. und diast. Blutdruck und Puls nach einmaliger Brevimytalinjektion (Dosierung 1–1,5 mg/kg/KG.)

konnten wir allerdings einen Blutdruckabfall feststellen, der beim Methohexital nie 20 mmHg überschritt, beim Propanidid sich zwischen 20 und 40 mmHg bewegte und beim Thiopental ebenfalls 20–40 mmHg betrug. Die Pulsregistrierung zeigte beim Brevimytal nur geringe Schwankungen, beim Thiopental eine Verlangsamung der Pulsfrequenz um 10%, beim Epontol eine Steigerung von etwa 25%. Elektrokardiographisch konnten wir bei allen drei Substanzen keine signifikante Änderung hinsichtlich Reizbildung, Erregungsausbreitung und Erregungsrückbildung feststellen.

Allergische Reaktionen: Beim Brevimytal haben wir auch bei wiederholter Injektion bisher keine allergischen Reaktionen feststellen können (Abb. 3).

In unseren drei Gruppen (je 50 Patienten) haben wir allerdings auch beim Thiopental und beim Epontol keinerlei allergische Reaktionen registriert. Bei früheren Narkosen mit Epontol sahen wir jedoch zwei schwere allergische Reaktionen in Form eines typischen anaphylaktischen Schocks, die aber beherrscht werden konnten.

Singultus und Venenschmerz konnten wir nur einmal bei einer Brevimytal-Kurznarkose feststellen. Niesen, Husten sowie Krämpfe und Defäkation haben wir nie beobachtet. Brechreiz und Erbrechen haben wir bei unseren 150 Patienten niemals bemerkt. Über Brechreiz haben Patienten nach Brevimytal bei unseren früheren Beobachtungen gelegentlich nur dann geklagt, wenn wegen des längeren operativen Eingriffes die Kurznarkose durch ein Inhalationsnarkotikum fortgeführt werden mußte. Leichtere Bewegungen der Muskulatur konnten wir nach Methohexitalgabe in 6% der Fälle beobachten. Die Patienten machten aber postoperativ keine Angaben über Muskelschmerzen. Wir konnten weder partiellen noch totalen Laryngospasmus bei unserem Patientengut unter Kurznarkose registrieren.

Die Aufwachzeit bei Kurznarkosen nach Brevimytal und Epontol betrug durchschnittlich 30–50 sec, die kürzeste 10 sec, sowohl bei Brevimytal wie Epontol, die längste bei Brevimytal 120 sec und bei Epontol 90 sec. Beim Thiopental wachten die Patienten frühestens in 60 sec auf, und die längste Aufwachzeit betrug 300 sec.

Erholungsphase: Nach dem Aufwachen aus der Brevimytal- und Epontolkurznarkose erholten sich die Patienten sehr schnell, sie konnten in ca. 2–3 min aufstehen, waren dann zeitlich und örtlich gut orientiert, und spätestens nach 15 min waren neurologische Tests (Romberg, Finger-Finger und Finger-Naseversuch) negativ, so daß wir die ambulanten Patienten nach durchschnittlich 45 min entlassen konnten, allerdings nur in Begleitung.

Beim Thiopental vermochten die Patienten dagegen erst nach 6–8 min aufzustehen, und neurologische Fehlleistungen bei nicht seltenem Nachschlaf waren noch nach 20 min zu registrieren. Entlassen konnten diese Patienten frühestens nach 60–80 min wiederum nur in Begleitung werden.

Über Schwindelgefühl und Benommenheit haben unsere Patienten nach Brevimytal und Epontol nicht geklagt. Bei Thiopental gaben etwa 20% der Patienten ein gewisses Unsicherheitsgefühl an.

Psychische Veränderungen: Unsere mit Brevimytal narkotisierten Patienten waren im Vergleich zu Epontol mehr in einer depressiven Stimmungslage, vereinzelt kam es bei einigen sogar zum Schluchzen bis zum Weinen. Solche psychischen Veränderungen zeigten sich bei den Patienten bis maximal 10 min nach dem Aufwachen. Danach war das psychische Verhalten der Patienten völlig unauffällig.

Die mit Propanidid narkotisierten Patienten dagegen waren fast immer euphorisch. Beim Thiopental konnten wir eine wesentliche Änderung der Stimmungslage nach der Narkose nicht beobachten.

Zusammenfassung

Als Ergebnis unserer vergleichenden Beobachtungen zwischen Methohexital, Propanidid und Thiopental als i.v. Kurznarkotica können wir folgende Vorteile des Methohexitals gegenüber dem Thiopental feststellen:

1. stärkere und kürzere Wirkung
2. kürzere Einschlafzeit
3. geringere Atem- und Kreislaufbelastung
4. schnellere und gute Erholung, kein Nachschlaf
5. kürzere Aufwachzeit
6. schnellere Straßenfähigkeit

Gegenüber Epontol möchten wir bei Methohexital

1. geringere Kreislaufveränderungen und
2. das Fehlen von allergischen Reaktionen

als positiv registrieren. Allerdings ist wohl die Aufwachphase nach Epontol-Kurznarkosen für den Patienten etwas angenehmer.

Auch mit Methohexital dürfte die Suche nach einem idealen Kurznarkotikum nicht abgeschlossen sein. Wegen seiner geringen Nebenwirkungen im Vergleich mit anderen i.v. Kurznarkotica kommt es aber den Forderungen, die wir an ein solches stellen, sehr nahe.

Summary

As the result of our comparative observations on methohexital, propanidide, and thiopental as intravenous short-term anaesthetics, the following advantages of methohexital over thiopental were extablished:

1. stronger and shorter-lasting effect
2. more rapid sleep induction
3. lower load on respiration and circulation
4. more rapid and full recovery, no after-sleep
5. shorter arousal time
6. more rapid recovery of street safety.

As compared with Epontol, methohexital

1. produces less pronounced circulatory alteration
2. does not give rise to allergic reactions.

These properties may be registered as advantages. However, the arousal phase following Epontol short-term anaesthesia seems to be somewhat more agreeable for the patient.

With methohexital, the search for an ideal short-acting anaesthetic is not concluded. Due to the very mild side-effects it produces as compared with those of other intravenous short-acting anaesthetics, it very nearly fulfils the requirements for such a preparation.

Kurznarkosen mit Methohexital

Von **F. Elchlepp**

Aus der Anaesthesie-Abteilung (Chefarzt: Dr. CH. LEHMANN)
der Chirurg. Klinik und Poliklinik (Direktor: Prof. Dr. G. MAURER)
am Klinikum rechts der Isar der Technischen Universität München

Um das Prädikat Kurz- bzw. Ultrakurznarkotikum konkurrieren heute im wesentlichen 3 Präparate, von denen das Ketamine diese Bezeichnung wegen des langen Nachtschlafes nicht beanspruchen kann. Um das Propanidid entstanden in den letzten Monaten Diskussionen, die viele Anaesthesisten veranlaßten, seinen Gebrauch einzuschränken oder einzustellen. Allein die Tatsache, daß es jetzt in Kombination mit einem Antiallergikum empfohlen wird, mindert seinen Wert als Kurznarkotikum erheblich [9]. Dagegen erwies sich Methohexital nach unseren und nach den Erfahrungen anderer als weitgehend problemlos und kommt den Idealforderungen an ein solches Präparat nahe [1, 2, 3, 6, 7, 11, 15, 16].

Allerdings hat auch dieses Mittel Nebenwirkungen wie Singultus, unwillkürliche Muskelbewegungen, kurzzeitige Apnoe und geringen Blutdruckabfall [1, 2, 3, 6, 11, 12, 14, 16]. Alternativpräparaten haften jedoch zum Teil dieselben, zum Teil andere, gravierendere Nachteile an, ohne gleichzeitig die Vorzüge von Methohexital zu bieten. Außerdem lassen sich die beschriebenen Nebenwirkungen durch langsame Injektion [3, 15, 16], Repetitionsdosen und durch Kombination mit Lachgas-Sauerstoff einschränken. Weder nach unseren Erfahrungen, noch nach Literaturberichten erreichen sie kritisches Ausmaß.

Demgegenüber stehen wesentliche Vorteile:

Methohexital wirkt nicht parasympathikomimetisch [3, 7, 8, 15, 17], läßt seinen Gebrauch bei Asthmatikern [2], Bronchitikern [3, 8] und digitalisierten Patienten also günstig erscheinen. Es zeichnet sich bei versehentlicher paravenöser Injektion durch geringe Gewebsirritation aus [3, 6, 8, 12, 19].

Übelkeit oder Erbrechen werden kaum ausgelöst [11, 12, 14, 16, 17].

Methohexital wirkt nicht hämolytisch [19], belastet Leber und Niere nur in geringem Maß [4, 5, 8, 17] und verursacht keine Stimulation des schwangeren Uterus [18].

Bei Patienten, die eine Kurznarkose erhalten, sind detaillierte Informationen über den Gesundheitszustand selten vorhanden. Auch die Anamnese gibt oft nur ungenügenden Aufschluß. Damit gewinnen die vorher genannten Eigenschaften unter Umständen besondere Bedeutung.

Die wesentlichsten Vorteile, die Methohexital bei Kurznarkosen bietet, sind das rasche Wiedererlangen des Bewußtseins, die kurze Erholungszeit mit fehlender Nachschlafneigung und die schnelle Rückkehr der Koordination [4]. Wie Frau DARBOVEN schon berichtete, sind Reaktionszeit und optische Fusion nach 30 min wieder normal. Dies ist gerade für ambulante Patienten wichtig, weil sie möglichst rasch straßenfähig sein sollen.

Bei Ambulanten ist eine Beeinträchtigung der schnellen Erholung durch unsachgemäße Prämedikation zu vermeiden. Scopolamin oder Morphinderivate sind wegen ihrer lang anhaltenden sedierenden Eigenschaften ungeeignet. Als neutralstes Mittel bewährt sich Atropin [12].

Da Methohexital – wie alle Barbiturate – keinen analgetischen Effekt hat, empfiehlt es sich, zusätzlich ein Lachgas-Sauerstoff-Gemisch zu geben. Erholungszeit oder Nachschlafneigung werden dadurch nicht beeinflußt, da Lachgas schnell wieder abflutet.

In den Jahren von 1966 bis 1969 wurden an der Anaesthesie-Abteilung des Klinikums rechts der Isar der Technischen Universität München 24483 Kurznarkosen bis zu einer halben Stunde Dauer mit Methohexital durchgeführt (Tab. 1).

Die Tabelle gibt Aufschluß darüber, auf welche Fachgebiete sich die einzelnen Betäubungen verteilen.

Um unsere Erfahrungen und unser Vorgehen darzulegen, möchte ich vor allem die Gruppen behandeln, die einen besonders hohen Prozentsatz an poor-risk-Fällen aufweisen.

Elektroreduktionen, Angiokardio- und Koronararterio-Graphien, Herzkatheter und Schrittmacherwechsel werden an Kranken durchgeführt, deren kardiale und Kreislauf-Verhältnisse am Rand der Dekompensation stehen. Bei den meist tachykarden bzw. tachyarrhytmischen Patienten, die einer Elektroreduktion unterzogen werden, verzichten wir auf jede Prämedikation.

Vor Kontrastdarstellungen des Herzens erhalten die Kranken Morphium-Scopolamin, dessen Wirkung wir als zufriedenstellend empfinden. Die in der Literatur beschriebene, durch diese Präparate ausgelöste Unruhe nach Brevimytal [10] wurde von uns nicht beobachtet. Zur Narkose verabreichen wir 60–80 mg Methohexital. Da diese Patienten fast immer eine verlängerte Kreislaufzeit haben, gerät man wegen des verzögerten Einschlafens unter Umständen in Versuchung, nachzuinjizieren. Die Einschlafzeit wird dadurch jedoch nicht verkürzt, das Aufwachen dagegen erheblich verzögert. Bei Injektion der genannten Dosen sind die Kranken nach 3–5 min wieder wach und voll ansprechbar.

Unter den Patienten, die sich einer Bronchoskopie unterziehen, befindet sich ebenfalls ein hoher Prozentsatz stark vorgeschädigter und alter Kranker

Tabelle 1. *Kurznarkosen mit Methohexital in den Jahren von 1966–1969*

Fachgebiet	1966	1967	1968	1969	Summe	Anwendung
Geburtshilfe		2220	2036	1764	6020	Durchtrittsnarkosen, Betäubungen zu Episiotomie-nähten
Gynäkologie	1293	1106	1105	984	4488	Abrasionen, Narkoseuntersuchungen
HNO	1048	1176	1439	1464	5127	Adenotomien, Tonsillektomien, Oesophago-Laryngo-Bronchoskopien
Thoraxchirurgie	1117	1170	1200	1146	4633	Bronchoskopien
Chirurgie	365	440	461	567	1833	kurzdauernde chirurgische Eingriffe
Röntgendiagnostik	101	235	430	578	1344	Angiographien, Bronchographien
Kardiologie	81	84	123	197	485	Elektroreduktionen, Angiokardio- und Koronar-Arterio-Graphien.Herzkatheter,Schrittmacherwechsel
Urologie	21	73	100	229	423	Cystoskopien, Elektroresektionen
Neurochirurgie	3	14	56	57	130	kurze neurochirurgische Eingriffe
	4029	6518	6950	6986	24483	

mit Störungen der Atmung und Beeinträchtigung der Herzleistung. Etwa die Hälfte der Bronchoskopien wird ambulant durchgeführt.

Die Prämedikation erfolgt mit Atropin und Silomat, um den postbronchoskopischen Reizhusten zu dämpfen. Je nach Zustand des Kranken geben wir 80–150 mg Methohexital, relaxieren mit 40–60 mg Succinylbischolin und verabfolgen Sauerstoff zunächst über die Maske, später über das Beatmungsbronchoskop. Auch hier sahen wir keine ernsten Komplikationen, die dem Methohexital anzulasten wären [3, 15].

Als besonderer Vorteil erweist sich die schnelle und vollständige Rückkehr des Bewußtseins, da gerade lungengeschädigte Patienten im Nachschlaf so flach atmen können, daß sie in die Hypoxie geraten.

Das Gleiche gilt für Kranke, die bronchographiert werden und bei denen aktives Abhusten besonders erwünscht ist.

Der Gruppe der Gefährdeten gehört auch das Kind unter der Geburt an, das anläßlich der der Mutter verabfolgten Betäubung in Mitleidenschaft gezogen wird. Das hier angewendete Mittel sollte den Organismus des Neugeborenen mit seinen noch nicht voll ausgebildeten Organfunktionen und Kompensationsmechanismen möglichst wenig belasten und im Interesse seiner Lebensfrische so kurz wie möglich wirken. Methohexital erfüllt diese Forderungen weitgehend.

Tonsillektomien und Adenotomien bei Kindern werden in Methohexital-Lachgas-Sauerstoff-Narkose und Intubation durchgeführt [3, 12]. Vertiefung und Verlängerung der Anaesthesie können durch Nachinjektionen von 10–20 mg Methohexital erreicht werden, ohne daß sich die Erholungszeit wesentlich hinauszögert. Halothan wird nicht benötigt. Damit hat der Operateur die Möglichkeit, das Operationsgebiet mit Adrenalin zu unterspritzen.

Die Verträglichkeit des Präparates erwies sich als so zufriedenstellend, daß wir es als Mittel der Wahl für kurzdauernde Narkosen bei Kindern ansehen.

Insgesamt läßt sich sagen, daß sich Methohexital als Kurznarkotikum bewährte, weil es die für diese Betäubungsform erforderlichen Kriterien aufweist und die Nebenwirkungen unwesentlich sind.

Zusammenfassung

Nach einem kurzen Überblick über die Nebenwirkungen werden die Vorteile des Methohexitals speziell unter dem Blickwinkel seiner Verwendung als Kurznarkotikum (extrem kurze Erholungszeit) dargelegt. In diesem Zusammenhang wird Atropin als alleinige Prämedikation empfohlen, weil ihm kein sedierender Effekt anhaftet.

Anschließend erfolgt ein Erfahrungsbericht über Methohexital bei 24483 Kurznarkosen, der besonders auf Betäubung zur Bronchoskopie, bei kardiologischen Patienten (Kardioversion und Angiokardiographie), zur Tonsillektomie bei Kindern und auf die Durchtrittsnarkose eingeht.

Es wird festgestellt, daß Methohexital aufgrund seiner Eigenschaften als das beste Kurznarkotikum angesehen werden kann, das heute zur Verfügung steht.

Summary

After a brief review of the side-effects of methohexital, its advantages are discussed particularly under the aspect of its use as a short-acting anaesthetic (with an extremely short recovery time). In this context, atropine is recommended as the premedication, since it has no sedative effect.

Subsequently, a report is given on the experiences gained with methohexital in 24483 short anaesthesias with special regard to anaesthesia in bronchoscopy, in cardiological cases (cardioversion and angiocadiography), in tonsillectomy in children, and in anaesthesia during emergence of the foetal head.

With these properties we believe methohexital to be the best short-acting anaesthetic available at the present time.

Literatur

1. AYD, F. J.: Methohexital (Brevital): A New Anaesthetic for Electroconvulsive Therapy. Diseases Nervous System **22**, Nr. 7 (1961).
2. BARRY, C. T., RENNIE, G. G., MACPHERSON, M. M.: Methohexitone Sodium in Anaesthesia for Cystoscopy. Anaesthesia **17**, 176 (1962).
3. BAUER-EHNES, H., HÖLZINGER, J.: Zunehmende Verwendung des Methohexital. Vortrag gehalten anläßlich des III. Europ. Anaesthesiekongresses, Prag 1970.
4. BINKERT, E.: Vergleichende Untersuchungen über die Straßenverkehrstauglichkeit nach Thiopental- und Methohexital-Kurznarkosen. Schweiz. Med. Wschr. **91**, 1285 (1961).
5. BITTRICH, N. M., KANE, A. V. R., MOSHER, R. E.: Methohexital and its Effect on Liver Function Tests. A Comparative Study. Anaesthesiology **24**, 81 (1963).
6. CHRISTENSON, G. R., HEBERT, C. L., DRISCOLL, E. J.: Intravenous Barbiturate for Dental Outpatients. Anaesthesia **40**, 77 (1961).
7. CLERGET, O., COUINAUD, C.: Utilisation en Chirurgie générale du Méthohexital à propos de 250 Observations. Anesthésie, Analgésie, Réanimation **22**, 343 (1965).
8. COLEMAN, J., GREEN, R. A.: Methohexital. A Short-Acting Barbiturate. Anaesthesia **14**, 411 (1960).
9. DOENICKE, A., LORENZ, W.: Histaminfreisetzung und anaphylaktoide Reaktion bei i.v. Narkosen. Anaesthesist **19**, 413 (1970).
10. DUNDEE, J. W., MOORE, J.: The Effect of Scopolamine on Methohexital Anaesthesia. Anaesthesia **16**, 194 (1961).
11. EYRES, A. E., KERNKAMP, R.: Brevital Sodium (Methohexital) as an Anesthetic Agent in Electrocerebral Stimulation: A Résumé of Five Years of Clinical Experience. Int. J. Neuropsychiatry **1**, 149 (1965).

12. Hudson, M. W. P.: Methohexithone. Practitioner **194**, 421 (1965).
13. Körner, M.: Vergleichende Beobachtungen bei verschiedenen Narkotika für die Narkoseeinleitung zur Tonsillektomie der Kinder. Anaesthesist **14**, 321 (1965).
14. Koslin, A. J.: A Clinical Study of Intravenous Barbiturates in Oral Surgery. J. Alabama Dental Ass. **45**, 16 (1961).
15. Lehmann, Ch., Elgert, K., Weber, K.: Klinische Erfahrungen mit Methohexital-Kurznarkosen. Z. prakt. Anästh. **1**, 387 (1966).
16. Rectant, B. S.: Methohexital Sodium. Oral Surgery, Oral Medicine, Oral Pathology **13**, 1330 (1960).
17. Schumacher, M. J.: Brevital Sodium for Basal Anesthesia in Pediatrics. J. Am. Ass. Nurse Anesthetists. **30**, 283 (1962).
18. Sharpless, S. K.: Hypnotics and Sedatives. I. The Barbiturates. In: Goodman, L. S., Gilman, A.: The Pharmacological Basis of Therapeutics. pp 114 bis 115. N. Y. Macmillan Co. 1965.
19. Weyl, R., Baha Unal, Y. Alper: Clinical Evaluation of a New Ultrashort-Acting Oxygen Barbiturate for Intravenous Anesthesia. Surgery, Gynaecology and Obstetrics **107**, 588 (1958).

Present Trends in Dental Anaesthesia

By **John D. Buxton**

Consultant Anaesthetist to: The Guy's Group of Hospitals,
School for Dental Auxiliaries, New Cross, London, England

Introduction

The purpose of this short paper is to indicate some of the methods of anaesthesia and analgesia which are now used in dental practice in the United Kingdom and United States. It will be presumed that the dentist and the anaesthetist are two separate people, unless analgesic techniques are used when it will be understood that the dentist and anaesthetist are the same person.

Before proceeding with the indications for the methods, there are certain premises which are worth repeating. Firstly, dental anaesthetics are not given to save life. Secondly, they are not absolutely required for the performance of any dental procedure. Thirdly, the use of these methods will be influenced by, on the one hand, opinion based on argument and on the other, preference based on personal taste. Practitioners will therefore accept or reject the methods according to their persuasion.

In the last 30 years dental anaesthesia for the ambulant patient has evolved from the purely inhalational administration to the intravenous technique. Present day practice uses either the intravenous route or the combination of the intravenous and the inhalational methods.

Some patients require to be in a state of unconsciousness or unawareness during the performance of their dentistry. It is a need but not a necessity. This need, having been recognized, has encouraged the advances in analgesic techniques of the last few years.

The demand by patients for dentistry under some form of anaesthesia, analgesia or sedation, varies from practice to practice; it is influenced by the type of patient, his intelligence, his social level, and his distaste for dentistry. Similarly the persuasiveness of the dentist in favour of or in opposition to the use fo these techniques will influence the number of cases in which they are applied.

A number of drugs may be used in a variety of techniques. However simple methods, using small doses of the agents contribute to the patient's safety.

Indications for Anaesthesia or Analgesia

It has already been stated that the performance of dentistry cannot be regarded as necessary to save life, therefore the indications for the use of anaesthetics or analgesics for carrying it out can be no more than relative.

The cases presenting relative indications are:

1. Patients for whom dentistry is unacceptable.
2. Children who are uncooperative.
3. Spastics.
4. Educationally sub-normal patients.
5. Patients in whom local anaesthesia cannot be induced.
6. A further group or sub-group are those patients who require the performance of considerable programmes of dentistry but for whom multiple appointments are not possible.

Absolute Contraindications for Anaesthesia

The absolute contraindications for the administration of a general anaesthetic for the performance of dentistry occur in the following conditions:

1. The unprepared patient, that is the patient who has not fasted from food or fluid for 4 h.
2. The surgery unequipped for resuscitation, that is the facility for ventilating the patient with air or oxygen, and aspirating fluid or foreign bodies from the upper respiratory tract.
3. The absence of a third person at the time of the administration.

Relative Contraindications for Anaesthesia or Analgesia

The relative contraindications for the administration of anaesthetics or analgesics relate to any coincidental pathology in the patient.

Definitions

The transition from consciousness to surgical anaesthesia is not sharply demarcated. Just as surgical anaesthesia is recognized as occurring in several planes, so it may be considered that the transition between consciousness and surgical anaesthesia may also be progressive.

In the Fig. 1 the 3 main levels of sedation, amnesia, analgesia, are diagramatically related to each other; the overlapping that occurs is also indicated. As the patient is projected from consciousness to unconsciousness the progressive loss of response to the spoken word is shown. Similarly the glottic reflex is also gradually abolished. The blockade of painful impulses commencing at the onset of sedation becomes more effective as the patient approaches the level of surgical anaesthesia.

Each level will have a critical pain or stimulus value which when exceeded will produce a response by the patient at the time without mental recall after completion of the procedure. A greater stimulus will produce a response and recall.

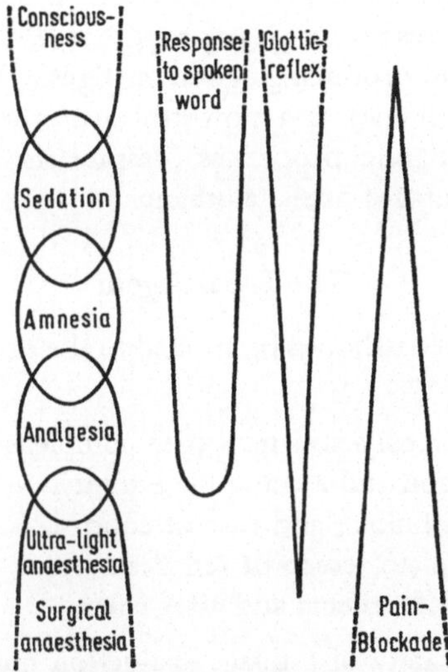

Fig. 1. The levels of diminished consciousness

Between consciousness and surgical anaesthesia there is not only a progressive loss of the protective laryngeal reflex, and the swallowing reflex, but also the ability to maintain a patent airway. In the management of all cases it must be assumed that the protective reflexes are not present, and vigilance in protecting the respiratory tract from the entry of fluid and foreign matter must be exercised. The airway, even though spontaneously patent in some cases, must be assiduously maintained at all times in all levels of unconsciousness.

The type of dentistry planned, whether producing little or no pain, as in the preparation of a simple occlusal cavity, or producing considerable pain, as in exodontia, will determine the level of unconsciousness to be selected.

Drugs

The drugs used in dental anaesthesia are classified according to their main pharmacological effect. For example methohexitone (Brietal) is considered an anaesthetic agent; it, however, possesses both sedative and amnesic properties and is claimed to be a weak analgesic. Propanidid (Epontol) is an intravenous anaesthetic agent exerting an extremely short effect; it exerts no analgesic effect. Diazepam (Valium) is a sedative with strong amnesic properties and in large doses, not used in dentistry, may produce anaesthesia. The inhalational agent halothane (Fluothane) is a powerful anaesthetic, and possesses no analgesic properties. Trichlorethylene (Trilene) is a volatile adjuvant producing good analgesia but poor anaesthesia. Methoxyflurane (Penthrane) is a powerful anaesthetic and is claimed to possess powerful analgesic properties, despite its slower induction it is claimed to have advantages over halothane.

The Ideal Agent

The following criteria should be applied to the drugs in use. Each agent should provide:

1. Production of unconsciousness with complete safety.
2. Peaceful induction and a tranquil recovery.
3. Simplicity of technique and ease of control.
4. Rapid and complete return of reflexes.
5. Freedom from side-effects and after-effects.

In evaluating the safety of a drug, distinction must be drawn between the dangers associated with the drug itself and the complications following errors in technique. For example, there are no recorded deaths attributable primarily to methohexitone, but fatalities have been recorded following the improper administration of this agent and resulting from errors in management.

The peaceful induction associated with intravenous administration relieves the patient of anxiety. Equally the patient's tranquillity during the recovery phase is marked and is reflected in those looking after him.

Simplicity of technique ensures safety; the more complicated the procedure the greater the chance of some being omitted or incorrectly carried out. Ease of control implies that the agents should be fast-acting, by virtue of their pharmacological properties and also by their route of administration. The intravenous route permits the effect of the drug to be observed in the arm-brain circulation time, that is about 20–25 sec after administration. Consequently if the length of time the drug produces its effect is short, intermittent doses may be given in order to maintain the desired level of unconsciousness.

For this technique, an open-vein is maintained by inserting and securing an intravenous needle in the arm and connecting it through a length of fine bore tubing to a syringe containing the anaesthetic or analgesic agent.

The inhalational route compares unfavourably with the intravenous in terms of speed. The gaseous and volatile agents are space occupying, and the tension of the agent tolerated by the respiratory tract determines the amount that can be presented to the lung alveoli and the concentration subsequently achieved in the bloodstream. The blood/gas solubility coefficient, and the oil/gas coefficients similarly determine the speed of induction and the potency of the volatile agents. These physical properties similarly influence rate of recovery.

The rapid and complete return of reflexes is desirable in those protecting the respiratory tract as well as those responsible for balance and locomotion. The patients are invariably out-patients and they must be able to walk from the surgery minutes after completion of their dentistry.

Any side-effects induced by a drug, particularly resulting in a disturbance of the physiology of the respiratory or cardiovascular systems should preclude its use. The normal therapeutic dose should produce no effect on these centres; there should be neither respiratory depression nor impairment of cardiovascular function.

Equally undesirable after-effects such as collapse, nausea, vomiting, or headache are unacceptable. Patients may accept these sequelae following surgery in hospital, but will not appreciate their occurrence following what to the patients has been the performance of dentistry under some form of light anaesthesia or sedation.

Development of Technique

The following factors influence the choice of technique:

1. The experience of the administrator.
2. The length of the procedure.
3. The intensity of the stimulus of the procedure.
4. The known history of the patient.
5. The training of the staff and the availability of resuscitative facilities.

The skilled administrator will in the light of his experience be able to anticipate the painful manoeuvres during the performance of the dentistry and adjust the patient's level accordingly. During the non-stimulating phases the patient may be allowed to lighten even to consciousness. For this purpose a single agent such as methohexitone given intermittently may be perfectly satisfactory.

When dentistry is prolonged, or the stimuli considerable, consideration must be given to the total dose of the agent likely to be administered. It may be desirable to minimize the hangover effect and the delayed recovery by the complementary use of local anaesthesia.

Aged patients on account of their lower BMR compared with younger patients, require less of all drugs to produce a given effect. Furthermore the barbiturates in larger doses tend to be less well tolerated by the elderly who sometimes complain of feeling befuddled for some hours after long procedures.

In adolescents and children the administration of methohexitone does not invariably produce quiescent operating conditions. The patients are seen to over-react to minor stimuli, and produce the so-called excitatory phenomena. Further incremental doses may worsen the response rather than lessen it. Full anaesthesia may be produced by giving excessively high doses but this should not be carried out in the dental surgery; the resulting respiratory and cardiovascular depression may be marked. Furthermore recovery time may be greatly prolonged.

These cases are satisfactorily managed by administering either complementary local anaesthesia or an inhalational agent. Unless the stimuli are of a high order the use of pre-mixed nitrous oxide and oxygen (Entonox), in equal proportions and administered nasally from a simple apparatus, such as the Latham (Longworth Scientific Instrument Co. Ltd., Abingdon, Berkshire, England), will suffice. Occasionally, as in the resistent patient, it will be necessary to use a volatile adjuvant such as halothane. This compound technique is associated with the maintenance of the open-vein for incremental doses of methohexitone.

Endotracheal intubation is seldom required and for the longer cases is undesirable owing to the increased morbidity associated with this manoeuvre. In patients whose airways are difficult to maintain, the introduction of a naso-pharyngeal tube may resolve the difficulty.

Compound technique; the patient is receiving fractional doses of a 1% solution of methohexitone from a 10 ml syringe connected to an indwelling needle through flexible tubing. The anaesthetic apparatus is delivering a 50% oxygen and nitrous-oxide mixture through a small nasal hood. The anaesthesist is in the position of "first assistant" opposite the dentist, and is able to maintain the airway by continuous support of the chin. He is able to provide a dry field by suitable positioning of the high-volume/low-vacuum aspirator tip, and so protect the patient's respiratory tract from the entry of fluid and foreign bodies. The anaesthesist's further responsibility is to position and change the plastic foam pack as necessary.

This technique of "four-handed" dentistry may be carried out on all types of conservation, and in selected oro-surgical procedures.

The dose of methohexitone is frequently recorded with reference to body weight. This is only true for the induction dose however. In practice consideration must be given to the time factor. The relationship of total dose of methohexitone to the time and weight is approximately 6 mg/kg for the first hour, and 9 mg/kg for the first 2 h. When an adjuvant, such as halothane, has been used this is reduced to 3 mg/kg and 6 mg/kg respectively.

Propanidid (Epontol) which is very much shorter in effect than methohexitone, may be used in the same way, with the same precautions. It has an application in the adolescent patient, the patient who is undergoing an extremely short procedure, for the very elderly and for the epileptic. It is a viscous solution; for the induction, 10 ml of the 5% solution is given. It is less satisfactory than methohexitone for the longer cases.

Diazepam (Valium), which is primarily an intravenous tranquilliser, has a marked amnesic property. In large doses which should not be administered in the dental surgery, it will induce anaesthesia. When it is administered together with local anaesthesia, extremely apprehensive patients will accept prolonged procedures with equanimity. This agent has been of inestimable value to the single-handed dentist. The dose is 5–10 mg given slowly; the total dose should not exceed 20 mg for an adult.

The JORGENSEN technique has been largely supplemented by the shorter and more predictable diazepam. The technique devised by JORGENSEN consists of a slow intravenous administration of pentobarbitone to the point of observable cortical depression followed by the intravenous administration of pethidine 25 mg and hyoscine 0.4 mg. The success of the technique depends on its use with good local anaesthesia, and the time available for the performance of dentistry is related to the patient rather than to the dose of the agents; the time is constant for a given patient. Patients often complain of feeling sleepy for several hours afterwards.

Influence of Disease

So far in the consideration of anaesthesia and analgesia, only the healthy patient has been discussed. The influence of disease upon the selection of a particular technique will be determined by the experience and opinion of the anaesthetist.

History

The way in which the information about the patient is elicited is as follows.

In the first case a simple "screening" history can be taken by the dentist. This will enable a broad decision to be made as to the patient's suitability for a particular technique. If the patient is accepted for general anaesthesia a full history should be taken by the anaesthetist embracing the following:

1. Previous illnesses and operations.
2. Present diseases or disabilities.
3. Previous anaesthetics.

4. History of allergy especially with regard to penicillin and other drugs.
5. Course of drugs taken during the last three years.
6. Smoking habits and alcohol intake.
7. Diseases associated with the immigrant population.
8. Pregnancy.

It is unlikely that careful history taking will fail to disclose some physical disability precluding anaesthesia which would have otherwise been discovered only by full physical examination.

Complications

Considering all complications during the anaesthetic and post-anaesthetically, the incidence is extremely low.

Laryngeal stridor or spasm occurs extremely rarely; it is invariably due to the passage of fluid or foreign bodies beyond the pack during the dental procedure. It is a failure of technique and not the result of the administration of the agent or agents. The treatment is to remove the cause.

It is fair to say that not one intravenous agent is more likely to produce this complication than any other.

Hiccoughs occur in a number of patients. They may or may not be associated with any alimentary disease; occasionally they have been observed in patients with hiatus hernia. The administration of atropine sulphate perhaps reduces this incidence. In most cases the condition passes off spontaneously.

Venous thrombosis at the site of the injection occurs irrespective of the agents administered or the length of time that they have been administered. In these cases reassurance is all that is necessary.

Pre-anaesthetic Instructions

It is implicit that the rule of fasting from food and fluid for four hours is given in writing to every patient. However not every child or adult will after this time have an empty stomach; but the majority will, and the chances of vomiting during or after the induction are consequently reduced.

A patient should furthermore be instructed to avoid driving a car or operating machinery on the day of the procedure. Finally the patient should be requested to leave the premises accompanied after treatment. This offers some safeguard to the euphoric patient following the use of diazepam, and to the drowsy patient following the JORGENSEN technique.

Summary

At the present time the use of methohexitone in conjunction with an inhalational technique provides a safe and satisfactory method of light general anaesthesia for the performance of most forms of dentistry carried out in the surgery on ambulant patients.

Zusammenfassung

Zum gegenwärtigen Zeitpunkt stellt die Anwendung von Methohexital in Verbindung mit einem Inhalationsverfahren eine ungefährliche und zufriedenstellende Methode der leichten Allgemeinnarkose für die Durchführung der meisten Arten von zahnärztlichen Eingriffen, die bei ambulanten Patienten in der Praxis vorgenommen werden, dar.

Methohexital, Thiopental und Propanidid in der Elektroschockbehandlung

Von **P. Rudolph**

Aus der Abteilung für Anaesthesiologie der Universität Würzburg
(Vorstand: Prof. Dr. K. H. Weis)

Die Elektroschockbehandlung besitzt in der Psychiatrie nach wie vor ihren festen Platz! Sie wird vor allem dort eingesetzt, wo bestimmte Psychosen – besonders solche des manisch-depressiven Symptomenkreises und der Schizophrenie – auf die übliche medikamentöse Therapie nicht befriedigend ansprechen. Obwohl die elektrische Auslösung des therapeutisch genutzten epileptischen Anfalls schmerzlos verläuft, stellt der Ablauf der Heilkrampfbehandlung für den wachen Patienten ein belastendes Erlebnis dar. Deswegen ging man dazu über, das Bewußtsein des Patienten für diesen Eingriff mittels einer Kurznarkose auszuschalten. Außerdem lassen sich hierbei typische Komplikationen der Elektroschocktherapie, nämlich Knochenbrüche, Distorsionen und Muskelzerrungen mit Succinylcholin weitgehend vermeiden.

Da die Elektroschockbehandlung nicht selten auch bei ambulanten Patienten durchgeführt wird, muß der Anaesthesist eine Narkoseform auswählen, bei der rasch die notwendige Tiefe erzielt wird und trotzdem nur ein kurzer Nachschlaf folgt. Dies läßt sich mit den kurzwirksamen Barbituraten Methohexital und Thiopental sowie dem Phenoxyessigsäurederivat Propanidid erreichen. Im folgenden soll über eigene Erfahrungen mit diesen Kurznarkotica berichtet werden.

In der Zeit vom 5. 6. bis zum 5. 11. 70 wurden in der Würzburger Universitätsnervenklinik bei 72 Patienten 263 Kurznarkosen anläßlich der Elektroschockbehandlung durchgeführt, wobei Methohexital 140mal, Thiopental 69mal und Propanidid 54mal verwendet wurde. Alter, Geschlechtsverteilung und zugrundeliegende Diagnosen sind als Mittelwerte in der 1. Tabelle aufgeführt.

Als Prämedikation erhielten alle Kranken ca. 30 min vor Narkosebeginn 0,5 mg Atropin. 90 Methohexitalnarkosen, 38 Thiopental- und 29 Propanididnarkosen wurden zusätzlich mit 1–2 ml Thalamonal vorbereitet. Die Narkosen wurden dann mit folgenden in Vorversuchen ermittelten und auf

Tabelle 1. *Alter, Geschlechtsverteilung und zugrundeliegende Diagnosen von 72 Patienten, bei denen 263 Kurznarkosen anläßlich der Elektroschockbehandlung durchgeführt wurden*

Anzahl	Alter	männlich	weiblich
72	39,5	30	42
Depression	Manie	Schizophrenie	sonstige
52	11	5	4

Gewichtsbasis errechneten Mengen eingeleitet, wobei bestimmte Injektionszeiten eingehalten wurden:

und zwar

1 mg/kgKG Methohexital in 12 sec
2 mg/kgKG Thiopental in 6 sec
6 mg/kgKG Propanidid in 24 sec.

Anschließend wurde zur Mitigierung des Elektrokrampfes 0,5 mg/kgKG Succinylcholin injiziert.

Zur Beurteilung des Narkoseablaufes dienten verschiedene Kriterien (Tab. 2): Die Einschlafzeit, definiert als die Zeit vom Beginn der Narkosemittelinjektion bis zum Verschwinden des Lidreflexes, erweist sich bei der Propanididgruppe am kürzesten. Thalamonal (in der Tabelle mit c. Th. bezeichnet) verkürzt sie in der Methohexital- und Thiopentalgruppe, nicht dagegen im Propanidid-Kollektiv.

Die Schlafdauer reicht vom Verschwinden des Lidreflexes bis zum Erwachen des Patienten aus der Narkose, wenn er seine Augen auf Anruf öffnen und gerichtete Augenbewegungen ausführen kann. Während die Zeiten für Methohexital und Propanidid eng beieinander liegen, schlafen die Patienten der Thiopentalgruppe länger. Thalamonal verlängert die Schlafdauer in allen drei Gruppen.

Tabelle 2. *Einschlafzeit und Schlafdauer in sec nach Kurznarkose mit Methohexital, Thiopental und Propanidid (Mittelwerte)*

		Methohexital	Thiopental	Propanidid
Einschlafzeit	s. Th.	73	84	52
(sec.)	c. Th.	67	63	52
Schlafdauer	s. Th.	351	384	353
(sec.)	c. Th.	426	455	390

Das Verhalten von Blutdruck und Puls ist in Tabelle 3 dargestellt. Der 1. Wert wurde vor Einleitung der Narkose bestimmt, der 2. beim Wiedereinsetzen der Spontanatmung, d. h. ca. 100 sec nach Auslösung des Elektroschocks und der 3. Wert beim Erwachen des Patienten aus der Narkose. Während die Pulsfrequenz in der Beobachtungsperiode praktisch konstant bleibt, erhöhen sich verübergehend systolischer und diastolischer Blutdruck bei allen Kollektiven.

Tabelle 3. *Verhalten von Blutdruck und Pulsfrequenz (Mittelwerte)*

	Methohexital		Thiopental		Propanidid	
	RR	Fr.	RR	Fr.	RR	Fr.
1.	128/81	102	125/82	92	128/79	96
2.	150/94	99	158/100	95	161/99	97
3.	133/84	101	136/87	95	137/85	98

Nebenwirkungen traten bei jeder Patientengruppe in unterschiedlichem Maße auf. Bei Methohexital- und Thiopentalnarkosen wurden die üblichen bei Barbituraten vorkommenden Nebenwirkungen, nämlich leichte motorische Unruhezustände, Singultus, Atemdepression nach zu rascher Injektion und Übelkeitserscheinungen beobachtet. Ernsthafte Komplikationen traten nicht auf. In der Propanididgruppe dagegen mußten neben banalen auch ernste Zwischenfälle registriert werden. Bei 2 Patienten kam es im unmittelbaren Anschluß an die Propanididinjektion zu schweren anaphylaktisch-allergischen Reaktionen, die zum Abbruch der Elektroschockbehandlung zwangen. Nach Gabe von 400 bzw. 300 mg Propanidid in 24 bzw. 15 sec fiel plötzlich der Blutdruck massiv ab und der periphere Puls war nicht mehr tastbar. Laryngo- und Bronchospasmus komplizierten die Situation bei jenem Patienten, welcher seit längerem an Asthma bronchiale leidet. Schließlich manifestierten sich an der Haut unterschiedlich ausgedehnte Erytheme, welche teilweise mit Quaddeln durchsetzt waren. Ödeme an den Oberlidern und am Larynx – hier mit Stridor einhergehend – vervollständigten das Bild des anaphylaktischen Schocks. Unter intensiver Therapie mit Corticosteroiden, Antihistaminica, Euphyllin und Plasmaexpandern bildete sich die bedrohliche Symptomatik innerhalb von 1–2 Std zurück. Spätfolgen traten nicht auf. Bemerkenswert ist, daß bei beiden Patienten anamnestisch eine allergische Disposition ausgeschlossen werden konnte. Eine vorherige Propanididinjektion hatte nur bei einem Kranken stattgefunden.

Neben den erwähnten klinischen Kriterien des Narkoseablaufes wurde bei einigen Patienten das Verhalten bestimmter Serumbestandteile, nämlich

Cholesterin, Ca, anorg. Phosphat, Gesamtbilirubin, Albumin und Gesamteiweiß, Harnsäure, Rest-N, Glukose, LDH, alk. Phosphatase und SGOT mit einem Autoanalyser gemessen. Dabei wurde die 1. Blutprobe vor Einleitung der Narkose, die übrigen 5, 10 und 20 min nach der Narkosemittelinjektion entnommen. In allen Fällen konnten bis auf eine mäßige Blutzuckererhöhung, die in der Propanididgruppe signifikant war, und einen leichten Abfall des Calcium-Spiegels keine nennenswerten Abweichungen vor den Ausgangswerten registriert werden.

Außerdem wurden mit dem Coulter-Counter Leukocyten, Erythrocyten, Hb, HK, HbE und mittleres Corpuscularvolumen der Erythrocyten bestimmt. Abgesehen von einem bei allen Narkosemitteln auftretenden, nicht signifikanten Anstieg der Leukocyten sowie einem geringgradigen Abfall der Erythrocyten ließen sich keine Änderungen von den Ausgangswerten nachweisen.

Die zahlenmäßige Auswertung eigener Kurznarkosen bei der Elektroschockbehandlung zeigt, daß die Art der Prämedikation einen deutlichen Einfluß auf die Narkosedauer hat. Thalamonal in der Prämedikation verkürzt geringfügig die Einschlafzeit, verlängert aber gleichzeitig die Schlafdauer und damit die gesamte Erholungszeit erheblich. Am ausgeprägtesten läßt sich dieser Effekt bei den Barbituraten nachweisen, während er bei der Propanididgruppe nicht ganz so deutlich in Erscheinung tritt. Da die zur Elektroschockbehandlung ausgewählten Patienten in der Regel unter dem Einfluß neuroleptisch und sedativ wirkender Psychopharmaka stehen, kann mit EICHLER und BÖHME die ausschließliche Prämedikation mit Atropin empfohlen werden, um die Vorteile der Kurznarkose voll ausnutzen zu können. In diesem Fall liegen die Zeiten für die Schlafdauer bei den untersuchten Kollektiven relativ nahe beieinander. Beim Vergleich mit den Angaben anderer Autoren zeigen die ermittelten Werte nur für Methohexital eine annähernde Übereinstimmung. LAWRENCE u. Mitarb. haben darauf hingewiesen, daß nach Injektion von 200–250 mg Thiopental (= 3 mg/kg KG) mit einer Schlafdauer von 11–15 min zu rechnen ist. Die eigenen Werte liegen bei einer Dosierung von 2,1 mg/kg KG entsprechend niedriger, erreichen jedoch nicht die Ergebnisse von Methohexital und Propanidid. Bis zum Aufwachen vergehen nach der Gabe von 250–500 mg Propanidid gemäß WEERTS, BECK u. MICHEL 3–5 min. Dabei handelt es sich jedoch nicht um Elektroschocknarkosen, bei denen der epileptische Anfall von einem Nachschlaf gefolgt wird, so daß sich zwangsläufig höhere Werte ergeben.

Während Propanidid bei den Einschlafzeiten am günstigsten abschneidet, unterscheiden sich Methohexital und Propanidid hinsichtlich der Schlafdauer nur wenig voneinander. Die weitere Erholungsphase, die bei der vorliegenden Untersuchungsreihe aus methodischen und technischen Gründen nicht verfolgt werden konnte, verläuft im Falle der Elektroschocktherapie anhand von Literaturangaben (Frank, Coleman, Eichler usw.) annähernd parallel.

Dagegen haben mehrere Autoren darauf hingewiesen, daß dem Thiopental eine deutlich längere Erholungsphase folgt. Diese Angaben stimmen nur bedingt mit den eigenen Untersuchungsergebnissen überein, weil die gesamte Erholungszeit nicht erfaßt wurde.

In bezug auf den Kreislauf verhalten sich die geprüften Kurznarkotica gleichartig. Nach dem Elektroschock steigt der systolische und diastolische Blutdruck infolge zentraler Stimulation an, während die Pulsfrequenz praktisch konstant bleibt. Die eigenen Ergebnisse lassen erkennen, daß Methohexital den zentral bedingten Blutdruckanstieg am stärksten dämpft, was bei Hypertonikern von Vorteil sein kann.

Die übrigen zum Narkoseablauf herangezogenen Kriterien zeigten keine wesentlichen Abweichungen zwischen den untersuchten Kollektiven.

Unter den beobachteten Nebenwirkungen heben sich die beiden anaphylaktischen Reaktionen nach Injektion von Propanidid deutlich von den übrigen, klinisch als harmlos zu bezeichnenden Komplikationen ab. Mehrere Autoren haben mittlerweile gleichartige Erfahrungen bei Propanididnarkosen beschrieben. Die Mehrzahl stimmt darin überein, daß hierbei möglicherweise Histamin eine kausale Rolle spielt. Nach Lorenz u. Doenicke muß besonders bei der Schußinjektion mit einer übersteigerten Histaminausschüttung gerechnet werden. Aus diesem Grund ist eine rasche Propanididgabe unter 20 sec unbedingt zu vermeiden. Umgekehrt darf jedoch nicht der Schluß gezogen werden, daß eine langsame Injektion über 20 sec allergische Reaktionen verhindert, was einer der beiden Fälle deutlich zeigt.

Aus dem Gesagten geht hervor, daß bei Anwendung von Propanidid

1. darauf geachtet werden sollte, in die Prämedikation grundsätzlich eine Antihistaminikum einzubeziehen,
2. auf eine Schußinjektion zu verzichten und
3. Allergiker sowie allergieverdächtige Personen auszuschließen.

Die üblichen Vorsichtsmaßnahmen wie Möglichkeit zur künstlichen Beatmung und zur Behandlung von Schockzuständen müssen selbstverständlich erfüllt sein. Seit im Jahre 1966 Currie u. Mitarb. nach Thiopentalinjektionen ebenfalls anaphylaktische Reaktionen beschrieben haben, muß der Anaesthesist auch bei derartigen Narkosen mit allergischen Komplikationen rechnen.

Zusammenfassung

Zusammenfassend darf festgestellt werden, daß alle drei Präparate bei der Elektroschockbehandlung eingesetzt werden können. Propanidid führt zu kürzesten Narkosen, es ist jedoch mit ernsten allergischen Komplikationen zu rechnen; Thiopental hat die längste Narkosedauer und Methohexital kommt den gewünschten Forderungen: *ausreichend tiefe Narkose bei kurzer Dauer* in seiner unproblematischen Anwendungsweise am nächsten.

Summary

In summary it may be stated that all three preparations can be employed in electroconvulsive treatment. Propanidide is the shortes-acting anaesthetic however, it may give rise to severe allergic complications. Thiopental anaesthesia has the longest duration, and methohexital, being most easy to administer, complies best with the requirements: *sufficient deepness and short duration of anaesthesia.*

Brietal bei 265 chirurgischen Notfällen

Von **J. P. Gauthier-Lafaye**, **M. Andres**, **J. Masson** und **J. M. Mascaro**

Département d'Anestésiologie, Strasbourg, France

Wir haben mit 265 Patienten einen Versuch durchgeführt, der das Ziel
hatte, den Nutzen von Brietal in der Notfallanaesthesie zu prüfen. Die
Notfallchirurgie stellt für den Anaesthesisten ein echtes Sondergebiet dar,
bei dem er mit viel Umsicht vorgehen muß. Er hat es dabei sehr oft mit
einem ihm unbekannten Patienten zu tun, dessen Vorgeschichte und dessen
vorangegangene Behandlungen er nicht kennt. Funktionsstörungen sind
manchmal verschleiert oder durch eine unter großem Zeitdruck durchgeführte Notfallbehandlung unvollständig erkennbar.

Aus all diesen Gründen muß der Anaesthesist über Medikamente verfügen, die die Herz- und Atemfunktion möglichst wenig beeinträchtigen,
auf die Ausscheidungswege nicht toxisch wirken und sehr schnell eliminiert
werden, um ein rasches Erwachen sicherzustellen. Es ist also kein Zufall,
daß bei diesen Narkosen Brietal eingesetzt wird.

Die pH-Stabilität der Lösung

Wir wollten zunächst die pH-Stabilität der Lösung überprüfen. Zu
diesem Zweck haben wir 500 mg Brietal in 50 ml destilliertem Wasser
gelöst. Eine Probe wurde bei 27° aufbewahrt, eine zweite bei 18° und eine
dritte bei Kühlschranktemperatur von 4°. Aus diesen drei Behältern wurden
Proben zur pH-Messung vom 1. bis zum 15. Tag entnommen (vgl. Tab. 1).
Die Tabelle zeigt, daß die pH-Änderungen im Laufe der Zeit unabhängig
von der Temperatur recht gering sind.

Obwohl das pH der Lösung bei jeder Temperatur, der die Probe aus-
gesetzt ist, konstant bleibt, sind wir doch der Ansicht, daß man sie zweck-
mäßigerweise bei Kühlschranktemperatur, d. h. bei 4° aufbewahren sollte.
Bei dieser Temperatur verhindert man das Angehen von Keimen, die
vielleicht zufällig hineingekommen sind.

Wenn man umgekehrt Flaschen mit 100 mg Inhalt benutzt, sind die
Veränderungen stärker ausgeprägt. Die pH-Messungen wurden mit einem
an einen Computer angeschlossenen Radiometer durchgeführt.

Tabelle 1. *Tabelle der pH-Veränderung einer Brietal-Lösung im Laufe der Zeit*

	1. Tag	2. Tag	3. Tag	4. Tag	5. Tag	6. Tag	7. Tag	8. Tag	9. Tag	10. Tag
Brietal										
B. 500 mg 27	10,531	10,414	10,408	10,402	10,389	10,376	10,359	10,357	10,342	10,326
B. 500 mg 18	10,520	10,484	10,469	10,451	10,428	10,411	10,406	10,404	10,399	10,388
B. 500 mg 4	10,541	10,502	10,488	10,462	10,459	10,438	10,436	10,429	10,424	10,420
B. 100 mg 27	10,410	9,695								
B. 100 mg 4	10,532	10,107								

Sterilität der Lösungen

Wenn man die Dosis von 500 mg in eine Flasche gibt, kann man annehmen, daß sich am Ende kein Bakterienwachstum im Behälter zeigt.

Wir haben regelmäßig nach der letzten Entnahme 1 cm³ des Präparates in der Flasche zurückgelassen und diesen Rest an das Hygienische Institut (Prof. LAVILLAUREIX) eingesandt. Es hat sich gezeigt, daß Lösungen, die zwischen 9 und 18 Tagen alt waren, keine Verunreinigungen aufwiesen. Die bakteriologische Kontrolle verlief stets negativ. Die Entnahmen müssen selbstverständlich unter den üblichen aseptischen Kautelen erfolgen.

Diskussion

Tabelle 2: Unter den 265 Fällen finden sich 88 Männer und 177 Frauen. Der Beginn der Prüfung mit gynäkologischen Notfällen erklärt das Mißverhältnis bei der Geschlechtsverteilung.

Tabelle 2. *Zahl der Narkosen*

nach Geschlechtern verteilt	
männlich	weiblich
88	177

Tabelle 3: In 88 Fällen wurde Brietal in einmaliger Injektion als alleiniges Narkotikum gegeben. In 177 Fällen wurde Brietal entweder allein mit Nachinjektionen oder in Kombination mit anderen Narkosemitteln verabreicht.

Tabelle 3. *Verteilung der Technik*

a) Kurzdauernde Allgemeinnarkose. Alleinige Brietalanwendung	88
b) Narkose, bei der Brietal nur zur Einleitung verwandt wurde	177

Tabelle 4: Diese Tabelle zeigt die altersentsprechende Aufteilung des Versuchs und die jeweils angewandte Technik. Wir sehen, daß die am häufigsten vorkommende Altersgruppe Erwachsene von 16 bis 50 Jahren umfaßt. Es sind 71% der Fälle.

Tabelle 5: Die Tabelle gibt die altersentsprechende Aufteilung der jeweils angewandten Technik wieder. So findet sich beim Kind vorwiegend die Kombination mit Fluothane. Beim Erwachsenen ist die häufigste Kombination Brietal plus Brietal-Lachgas. Sie findet sich in 75% der Fälle. In den restlichen 25% wurde Brietal mit einem anderen Präparat kombiniert.

Tabelle 4. *Verteilung nach dem Alter*

	Brietal allein	Brietal mit Nach-injektion + N_2O	Brietal + Kombina-tion	Gesamt	%
Unter 1 Jahr					
1–7 Jahre	1	1	12	14	6
8–15 Jahre	2	7	10	19	8
16–50 Jahre	55	77	49	181	71
50–70 Jahre	30	18		48	14
Über 70 Jahre			3	3	1

Tabelle 5. *Verteilung der Technik nach dem Alter*

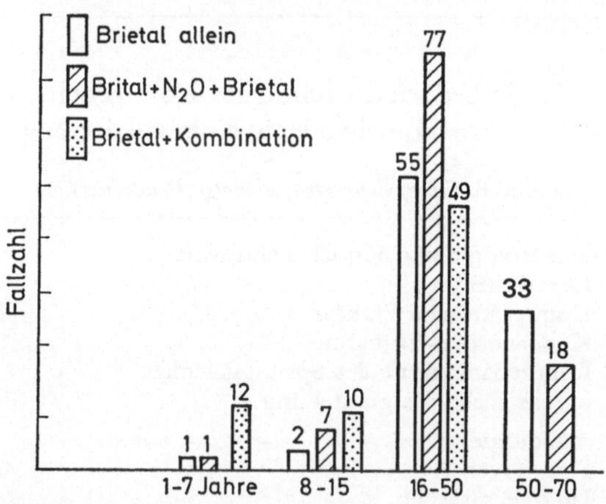

Tabelle 6: Wir sehen in dieser Tabelle, daß bei allen Kombinations-fällen die wiederholte Injektion plus Lachgas am häufigsten vorkommt (103 Fälle).

Tabelle 6. *Kombinationen mit Brietal*

Brietal + N_2O	103
Brietal + N_2O + Fluothane	47
Brietal + Méthoxyflurane	5
Brietal + Pheno + N_2O + Curare	4
Brietal + Pheno + Pentho + N_2O + Curare	18

Tabelle 7: Diese Tabelle befaßt sich mit dem Operationsrisiko. In 161 Fällen traf der Unfall gesunde Menschen. In 75 Fällen waren krank-hafte Veränderungen vorhanden. In 29 Fällen bestand ein Schockzustand;

es handelte sich dann darum, die Narkose während der Schockbekämpfung durchzuführen.

Tabelle 7. *Allgemeinzustand und Operationsrisiko*

I. Notfall bei gesunden Menschen	161
II. Notfall bei kranken Organsystemen	75
Herz-Kreislaufsystem	18
Atmung	39
Leber	7
Niere	6
Stoffwechselstörungen	5
Andere	
III. Notfall + Schock	29
Schock bei Gesunden	19
Schock bei Kranken	10

Tabelle 8 u. 9: Sie bedürfen kaum eines Kommentars. Sie stellen die Liste der Fälle dar, wo Brietal allein oder in Kombination angewandt wurde.

Tabelle 8. *Operationsarten, alleinige Brietalnarkose*

Traumatologie und Knochenchirurgie	
Luxationen	17
Dupuytren'sche Fraktur	2
Knochenspan-Entnahme	1
Röntgenaufnahme des Sprunggelenkes in maximaler Valgusstellung	35
Gynäkologie	
Kürettagen	10
Uterusrevisionen	2
Geburtshilfe	
Episiotomien	54
Bauch-Chirurgie	
Laparotomie wegen akutem Abdomen	3
Inkarzerierte Hernien	2
Appendektomie	39
Paraphimose	1
Hämorrhoidalthrombose	1
Neuroradiologie	
Neurochirurgie	
Radikotomie	1
Elektrokoagulation des Trigeminus	3
Andere	
Elektroschocks	20
Insgesamt	191

Tabelle 9. *Operationsarten, Narkoseeinleitung mit Brietal*

Traumatologie und Knochenchirurgie	10
Mehrfachverletzungen	
Osteosynthese bei offenen Frakturen	
Fraktureinrichtung	
Gynäkologie	31
Stielgedrehte Ovarialzyste	
Zervixriß	
Kürettagen, Bartholinitis	
Geburtshilfe	16
Uterusrevisionen	
Geburtshilfliche Maßnahmen	
Kaiserschnitt	
Bauchchirurgie	14
Perforiertes Ulcus	
Akute Appendizitis	
Darmverschluß	
Splenektomie	
Neuroradiologie	
Neurochirurgie	
Extradurales Hämatom	3

Insgesamt 74

Tabelle 10: Wir sehen, daß bei den Fällen, in denen Brietal allein oder in Kombination mit Lachgas gegeben wurde (191 Fälle), 91mal keine Prämedikation erfolgt ist. Dies war möglich, weil das Präparat keine vagotone Wirkung besitzt.

Tabelle 10. *Prämedikation – alleinige Brietalgabe oder Kombination mit N_2O*

Prämedikation		
Keine		91
Atropin allein		52
Atropin +	Pethidin	42
	Pethidin	
	+	
	Promethazin	6

Insgesamt 191

Tabelle 11: Wenn dagegen das Brietal mit einem anderen Narkosemittel kombiniert wurde, konnte auf eine Prämedikation nicht verzichtet werden.

Tabelle 11. *Prämedikation – Brietal, kombinierte Anwendung*

Prämedikation		
Keine		0
Atropin allein		52
Atropin +	Pethidin	20
	Pethidin + Promethazin	2

Insgesamt 74

Tabelle 12: In dieser Tabelle haben wir die Narkosedauer entsprechend der angewandten Technik dargestellt. Man kann daraus entnehmen, daß bei kurzdauernden Eingriffen von 5 min oder weniger Brietal allein als einmalige Injektion gegeben wurde.

Tabelle 12. *Narkosedauer*

	Brietal einmalige Injektion	Brietal + N_2O + nachinjiziertem Brietal	Brietal + N_2O + Fluothane	Brietal + Methoxyflurane	Brietal + Curare + Pheno + ...
5 min	70				
5–10 min	18	42			
10–15 min		45	4		
15–30 min		16	23		2
30–100 min			20	8	15
100–200 min					1
200–300 min					1

Tabelle 13: Diese Tabelle gibt noch deutlicher die Art der Kombination je nach der Operationsdauer wieder. So wird bei Eingriffen bis zu 5 min Brietal allein als einmalige Injektion angewandt. Bei länger als 5 min dauernden Operationen wurde meistens die Technik der wiederholten Injektion und der Kombination mit Lachgas verwendet. Von 10 min an erscheint die Kombination mit Fluothane und ab 15 min wird praktisch immer mit Fluothane kombiniert.

Tabellen 14 und 15: In diesen Tabellen haben wir die Dauer bis zum Erwachen nach der letzten Injektion festzustellen versucht. Bei einer einmaligen Gabe von Brietal wachen 90% der Patienten in 5 min auf. Wenn man wiederholte Injektionen gibt, so ist der Anteil an Fällen, die später als nach 5 min aufwachen, größer als wenn man mit Lachgas kombiniert. Die Kombination mit Lachgas macht eine Verminderung der Reinjektionen und ein früheres Erwachen möglich. Wir sehen, daß beim Vorliegen einer Niereninsuffizienz die Dosis herabgesetzt werden sollte, da sich sonst das Aufwachen sehr verzögert. Wenn man mit Fluothane kombiniert, erfolgt das Aufwachen etwas später.

Tabelle 13. *Angewandte Technik und Narkosedauer (bis 30 min)*

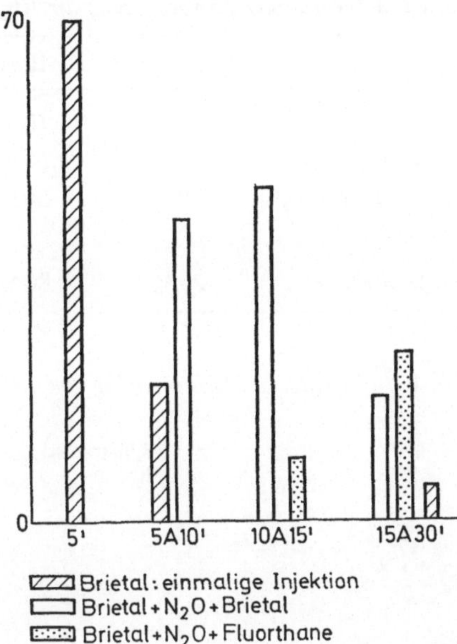

Tabelle 14. *Zeitdauer bis zum Erwachen in Abhängigkeit von der verabreichten Gesamtdosis*

	mg	< 5 min	5–10 min
Brietal einmalige Injektion	< 100	90 %	10 %
	100–150	64 %	36 %
Brietaleinleitung + Nachinjektionen	< 100	53 %	47 %
	100–150	37 %	63 %
	> 150	57 %	43 %

Tabelle 16: Die Tabelle zeigt, daß bei der Gabe von Brietal in angemessener Dosis (zwischen 0,5 und 1,5 mg/kg) die Schlafdauer zwischen 2 und 7 min beträgt. Wir sehen ferner, daß die Schlafdauer bei der gleichen Dosis die ein- bis dreifache Zeit betragen kann. Es besteht daher die Notwendigkeit, die nach dem Körpergewicht berechneten Standarddosierungen

zu verlassen und den Allgemeinzustand des Patienten zu berücksichtigen. Ein eiweißverarmter, anämischer, hypovolämischer Patient im Schockzustand hat alle Chancen, entsprechend später zu erwachen.

Wir sehen, daß zwei Patienten, die irrtümlich große Dosen erhalten hatten, verzögert aufwachten. Einer dieser Patienten war in einem schlechten Zustand.

Tabelle 15. *Zeitdauer bis zum Erwachen nach der letzten Injektion*

	5 min	10 min	länger als 15 min
Einmalige Dosis	90 %	10 %	
Einleitungsdosis + Nachinjektion	40 %	60 %	
Einleitung + Kombination mit N_2O	70 %	30 %	1 Fall von Niereninsuffizienz
Einleitung + N_2O + Fluothane	20 %	80 %	

Tabelle 16. *Verhältnis : Dosis in mg/kg zur Schlafdauer*

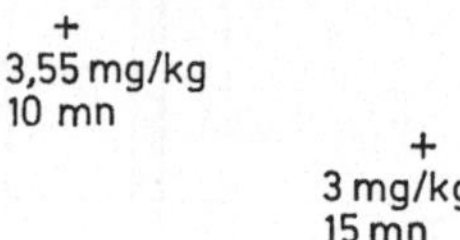

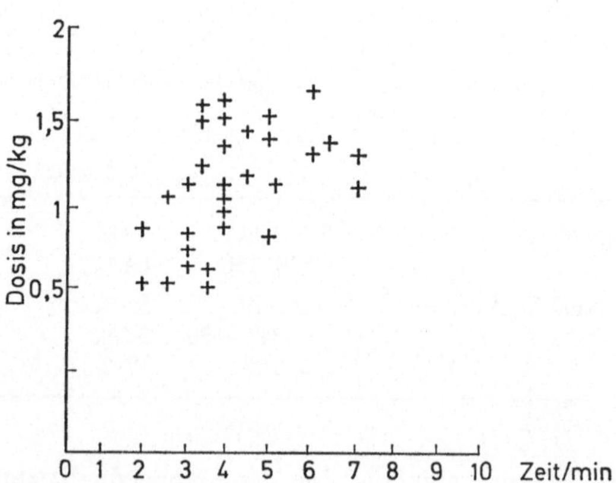

Tabelle 17: Diese Tabelle befaßt sich mit den Nebenwirkungen von Brietal auf das Herz-Kreislaufsystem. Die Blutdruckveränderungen wurden in 265 Fällen untersucht. Dasselbe gilt auch für die Herzfrequenz.

In 27 Fällen konnte der zentrale Venendruck geprüft werden.

In 10 Fällen wurde der Druck im rechten Ventrikel und ebenfalls in 10 Fällen der Druck in der Arteria pulmonalis gemessen. Eine vollständige elektrokardiographische Untersuchung wurde in 36 Fällen durchgeführt. Man kann aus dieser Untersuchung die bemerkenswerte Feststellung ableiten, daß die auftretenden Veränderungen ein geringes Ausmaß haben und nur kurzfristig anhalten. Sie treten ausschließlich in der Einleitungsphase auf.

Tabelle 17. *Nebenwirkungen auf das Herz-Kreislaufsystem*

	Blutdruck	Herz-frequenz	Zentraler Venen-druck	Druck im rechten Ventrikel	Druck in der A. pulmonalis	EKG
	265 Fälle	265 Fälle	27 Fälle	10 Fälle	10 Fälle	36 Fälle
Induktion	↗ 12 % → 51 % ↘ 37 %	↗ 47 % → 45 % ↘ 8 %	↘ 3 Fälle H_2O 1 %	Keine wesent-liche Änderung	Keine wesent-liche Änderung	Extra-systolen 1 Fall morpho-logisch völlig unver-ändert
Operation	N	N	N	N	N	N
Erwachen	N oder ↗	N oder ↗	N	N	N	N

Tabelle 18: Diese Tabelle zeigt das Verhalten des zentralen Venendrucks bei einigen der 27 diesbezüglich untersuchten Patienten.

Tabelle 19: Diese Tabelle beschreibt die 3 Fälle, bei denen ein Abfall des Venendrucks festgestellt wurde. Dieser Abfall hatte ein geringes Ausmaß und hielt nur kurz an.

Tabelle 20: Diese Tabelle befaßt sich mit den Wirkungen des Präparates auf die Atmung in Abhängigkeit von der angewandten Prämedikation. Die meisten Nebenwirkungen treten bei der Kombination Atropin-Analgetikum und Promethazin auf. Wie bei den Nebenwirkungen auf Herz und Kreislauf, sind auch diese Reaktionen von kurzer Dauer und finden sich nur in der Einleitungsphase. In 3 Fällen bestand allerdings während der gesamten Narkose ein Singultus.

Tabelle 21: Wir beabsichtigten, die Wirkung von Brietal auf den Elektrolythaushalt und die Blutgase zu untersuchen. Es wurden deshalb eine bestimmte Zahl von Tests bei 4 Patienten durchgeführt, damit die Ergebnisse vergleichbar sind. Sie können folgendermaßen interpretiert werden:

1. Die Patienten erhielten eine Narkose nur mit Brietal (Einleitung 2 mg/kg Körpergewicht) mit Reinjektionen je nach Bedarf. Eine Prämedi-

Tabelle 18. *27 Fälle, zentraler Venendruck während der Einleitung unverändert*

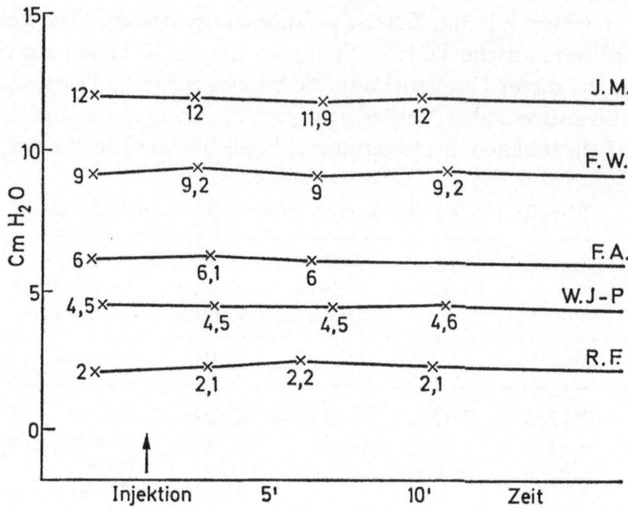

Tabelle 19. *3 Fälle mit verändertem zentralen Venendruck während der Einleitung*

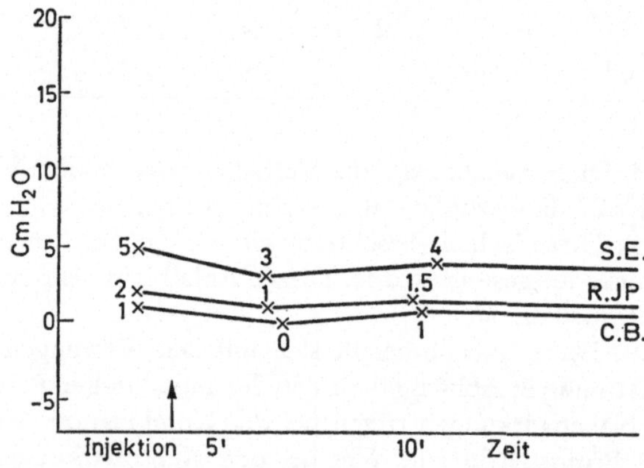

kation wurde nicht verabfolgt. Sie atmeten normale Luft. Die vier Operationen waren gleich schwer und umfaßten 3 Appendizitiden und einen Prolaps. Das Körpergewicht und das Alter waren verschieden. 3 Proben wurden abgenommen: eine vor der Injektion des Präparates, die zweite 5 min und die dritte 15 min nach der Injektion.

Mit der Operation wurde erst nach der ersten Probeentnahme begonnen, um jede Belastung des adrenergen Systems zu vermeiden, die die Ergebnisse verändern könnte. Es wurden bestimmt: der Harnstoff, der Blutzucker,

Tabelle 20. *Nebenwirkungen auf die Atemfunktion (265 Fälle)*

	Rhythmus	Amplitude	Apnoe	Husten	Schluckauf	Laryngospasmus
Einleitung Atropin	↘	↘	21	2	8	1
Atropin + Analgetikum	↘	↘	53		8	
Atropin + Analgetikum + Promethazin	↘	↘	70	3	14	
Operation					7	
Erwachen					3	1

das Natrium, das Chlorid, das Kalium, die Osmolarität, PO_2, Gesamt-PCO_2, SaO_2, pH. Wir sehen, daß die Veränderungen dieser Parameter recht unbedeutend waren. Es ist allerdings festzuhalten, daß es in allen Fällen und regelmäßig zu einem Blutzuckeranstieg kam.

Die Untersuchung der Wirkung von Brietal auf das Elektroenzephalogramm wurde nach der Injektion von 60 mg (1 mg/kg Körpergewicht) innerhalb von 10 sec durchgeführt.

1. Aufzeichnung: Die Kurven zeigen am Anfang eine Grundaktivität mit Alphawellen bei einer Frequenz von 9–10 c/s, mit mittlerer Voltage, normaler Verteilung, unregelmäßiger Modulation, wobei sie von bilateralen Thetawellen ohne Seitenbevorzugung überlagert oder unterbrochen werden.

2. Aufzeichnung: Vom Ende der Injektion an verlangsamen sich die Ausschläge und es kommt zum Auftreten einer ausgeprägten, langsamen Theta- und Delta-Aktivität von hoher Voltage, polymorph mit einem anterioren und temporalen Übergewicht. Diese langsame Deltaaktivität überlagert die Alphafrequenzen und die schnellen Rhythmen. Es tritt keine nennenswerte Veränderung der Atem- oder Pulsfrequenz ein.

3. Aufzeichnung: Diese polymorphe, generalisierte, langsame Aktivität bleibt bis 2 min nach Beendigung der Injektion bestehen und nimmt dann immer mehr ab. Eine Geräuschstimulierung führt zum Wiederauftreten der Alpha-Aktivität, während die langsamen Rhythmen blockiert sind.

4. Aufzeichnung: Die langsame Aktivität verschwindet drei Minuten nach Beendigung der Injektion vollständig. Nach einer weiteren Minute nennt der Patient auf Anruf seinen Namen und öffnet und schließt die Augen.

Tabelle 21

	L . . . 12 J. – 38 kg Appendizitis			M . . . 40 J. – 80 kg Appendizitis			S . . . 11 J. – 40 kg Appendizitis			B . . . 66 J. – 45 kg Prolaps		
	1	2	3	1	2	3	1	2	3	1	2	3
Harnstoff	0,32	0,34	0,33	0,36	0,34	0	0,30	0,30	0,30	0,26	0,26	0,27
Blutzucker	1	1,15	1,20	1,30	1,45	1,48	0,95	1,15	1,20	0,85	0,95	1
Na	135	135	135	144	135	140	138	135	134	142	144	
K	4,3	4,6	4,6	4,9	4,6	4,6	4,2	4	4	3,9		3,4
Cl	95	98	97	108	102	103	103	102	102	109		112
Osmol.	275	278	277	297	285	290	288	280	282	285		287
PO_2	89	90	89	75	74	80	90	92	90	79	80	82
PCO_2	41	40	40	41	40	42	38	35	36	32	34	31
CO_2 total	55	56	56	58	57	59	57	58	56	19,5	23	24
SaO_2	90	91	89	80	82	85	91	92	91	95,1	98,3	97
pH	7,38	7,39	7,39	7,41	7,39	7,38	7,38	7,37	7,39	7,40	7,42	7,45
Ca							1		2			

Narkosen mit Methohexital allein: — keine Prämedikation
— Brietal 2 mg/kg Körpergewicht
— Nachinjektion nach Bedarf

1 = vor der Injektion
2 = 5 min nach der Injektion
3 = 15 min nach der Injektion

Zusammenfassung

Das Brietal ist ein ultrakurz wirkendes Narkotikum, das das Herz-Kreislauf-System kaum beeinflußt und nur ganz kurz auf die Atmung und das Gehirn einwirkt. Seine Stabilität in gelöster Form gestattet seine Verwendung noch 14 Tage nach dem Ansatz. Die bei der Anwendung beobachteten Nebenwirkungen sind minimal, weisen aber darauf hin, daß das Präparat nur von Fachleuten benutzt werden sollte, die über die Möglichkeit einer Sauerstoffbeatmung verfügen.

Das Brietal ist ein beachtenswertes Mittel, das in der Anaesthesiologie sehr gute Dienste leistet.

Summary

Brietal is an ultrashort-acting anaesthetic. It hardly influences the cardiovascular system and affects respiration and brain only for a very short period of time. The substances shows a high degree of stability when dissolved. It may be used even a fortnight after the solution has been prepared. No more than minimum side-effects have been observed. Nevertheless, they indicate that it should only be used by experienced persons and when facilities for oxygen supply are available.

Brietal is a most remarkable preparation and may prove exceedingly useful anaesthesiology.

Methohexital in Risikofällen

Von **B.** und **G. Landauer**

Aus der Anaesthesie-Abteilung (Chefarzt: Dr. Ch. Lehmann)
der Chirurg. Klinik und Poliklinik (Direktor: Prof. Dr. G. Maurer)
am Klinikum rechts der Isar der Technischen Universität München

Der ständig wachsende Anteil der Alterschirurgie, die sprunghafte Zunahme schwerer Traumatisationen und die vorwiegend durch schonende Narkosetechniken bedingte Ausdehnung operativer Eingriffe konfrontieren den Anaesthesisten mit einer Vielzahl von Risikofällen.

Da diese Kranken in bezug auf ihre Belastungsmöglichkeit eine mehr oder minder unbekannte Größe darstellen, sind an ein zur Narkose-Einleitung und -Aufrechterhaltung verwendetes, intravenös gegebenes Anaesthetikum strenge Forderungen zu stellen:

1. schneller Wirkungseintritt und ausreichende Wirkungsstärke,
2. gute Steuerbarkeit,
3. kurze Wirkungsdauer,
4. geringe Kumulation,
5. weitgehende Verträglichkeit mit anderen im Rahmen der Allgemeinbetäubung verwendeten Präparaten,
6. unbedeutende oder fehlende Nebenwirkungen auf die bei gefährdeten Patienten meist am Rande der Kompensation stehenden vitalen Systeme,
7. geringe Belastung der Stoffwechselorgane und
8. Fehlen einer Uterusirritation sowie einer negativen diaplazentaren Beeinflussung des Kindes im Rahmen der geburtshilflichen Anaesthesie.

Diese acht Forderungen erfüllt das ultrakurzwirkende Oxybarbiturat Methohexital weitestgehend. Wir verwenden das Präparat auch in Risikofällen zu Kurznarkosen, zur Einleitung und zur kurzfristigen Narkosevertiefung.

In der geriatrischen Anaesthesie stellen bereits bestehende cardiovaskuläre Veränderungen wie Rechts-Linksherz-Insuffizienzen, Hypertonus, allgemeine Gefäßsklerose, chronisch kompensierter Volumenmangel, Ventilationsstörungen teils obstruktiven, teils restriktiven Charakters mit entsprechenden Blutgasveränderungen sowie altersbedingte degenerative Parenchymschäden bedeutende Faktoren dar, zu denen sich die durch die jeweilige Grundkrankheit hervorgerufenen Störungen addieren. Diese

Polymorbidität zwingt uns, wie SCHAUDIG formulierte, jeden alten Kranken a priori als Problempatienten zu betrachten.

Bei diesen Fällen ermöglichen bereits geringe Methohexitaldosen ein rasches, subjektiv angenehmes und störungsfreies Einschlafen. Exzitationserscheinungen wie Husten, Niesen, Singultus und unkoordinierte Muskelzuckungen können, wie DUNDEE u. Mitarb. zeigten, durch eine analgetische Prämedikation auf ein Minimum reduziert werden. Zu einer längeren Narkoseaufrechterhaltung läßt sich jedes beliebige Anaesthetikum verwenden.

Bei der Neuroleptanalgesie ersparen geringe Methohexitaldosen unangenehme Erinnerungen an den Intubationsvorgang.

Beim behandelten oder unbehandelten Hypertoniker werden gefährliche Blutdruckabfälle infolge der geringen Kreislaufbeeinflussung vermieden.

Die geringe Affinität dieses Anaesthetikums zum Körperfett bedingt im Gegensatz zu anderen Barbituraten ein rasches Absinken des Plasmaspiegels und ein schnelles, „overhangloses" oder wie es von französischen Autoren bezeichnet wird „sauberes Aufwachen" (netteté du reveil). Auf diese Weise werden postnarkotische Koordinationsstörungen und Ateminsuffizienz, Komplikationen, die einen günstigen postoperativen Verlauf nur allzu häufig in Frage stellen, vermieden.

Bei der Anaesthesie Schwerverletzter und Polytraumatisierter verdient, von der speziellen Problematik einzelner Verletzungen abgesehen, das Schockgeschehen mit seinen metabolischen und organischen Veränderungen besondere Aufmerksamkeit. Beim Schockierten genügen schon geringe Methohexitaldosen zur raschen Narkoseeinleitung. Sie können den Verzicht auf das vielfach bradyarrhythmisch wirkende Succinylcholin zur endotrachealen Intubation ermöglichen. Das Anaesthetikum trägt weder zur Schockverstärkung durch vermehrte Katecholaminausschüttung noch zu einer, bei anderen Barbituraten häufig beobachteten, oft deletären Durchbrechung einer bestehenden kompensatorischen Kreislaufzentralisation bei.

Die von mehreren Autoren beschriebenen parasympathikolytischen Eigenschaften erübrigen die in diesen Fällen unter Umständen problematische Atropin-Prämedikation und beugen einem durch Aspiration hervorgerufenen Mendelsson-Syndrom durch Bronchodilatation vor. Die Belastungen von Leber und Niere im Schock durch Abbau und Ausscheidung sind gering. Die rasche Wiederkehr der vitalen Schutzreflexe trägt auch bei diesen Kranken zum komplikationslosen postnarkotischen Verlauf bei.

Im Rahmen der neurochirurgischen Anaesthesie ist Methohexital bei Risikofällen sowohl zur Durchführung kurzer diagnostischer Eingriffe als auch zur Narkoseeinleitung längerdauernder Operationen geeignet. Weitgehende Kreislaufstabilität ermöglicht die gerade in diesem Spezialgebiet notwendigen extremen Operationslagerungen des Patienten. Das bereits beschriebene, schnelle Wirkungsende gestattet schon frühzeitig eine für die weitere Therapie wesentliche Beurteilung des Operationserfolges. Das Fehlen von postnarkotischem Erbrechen, Husten, und sonstigen Unruhezuständen vermeidet gefährliche Hirndruckanstiege.

Für Kranke mit Störungen der Atemfunktion besonders obstruktiven Charakters, bei denen eine Barbiturateinleitung bisher kontraindiziert schien, stellt Methohexital durch seine bronchodilatatorische Wirkung eine deutliche Bereicherung des Anaesthetika-Spektrums dar. Die in einigen Fällen beobachtete, kurz dauernde, zentrale Atemdepression braucht bei dem in der Regel intubierten und kontrolliert beatmeten Patienten nicht als ein Nachteil des Präparates angesehen zu werden.

Das rasche Erwachen mit frühzeitigem Einsetzen einer ausreichenden Spontanatmung im Verein mit der Fähigkeit, aktiv abzuhusten, verhindert Hypoventilation, Sekretretention und Bildung von Atelektasen.

Zur Narkose bei bronchoskopischen Untersuchungen meist älterer, cardial und pulmonal geschädigter Kranker verwenden wir das Mittel seit Jahren. Neben den bereits angeführten positiven Eigenschaften erweist sich die schnelle Straßenfähigkeit der vorwiegend ambulanten Patienten von Vorteil.

Bei Kranken mit Einschränkung der Leberfunktion kann das Anaesthetikum im Gegensatz zu vielen anderen Barbituraten, obwohl es in der Leber abgebaut wird, verwendet werden. Eine Studie von BITTRICH u. Mitarb. zeigt, daß klinische Dosen die Funktion des geschädigten Organs nur geringfügig beeinträchtigen.

Oligurischen und anurischen Patienten kann Methohexital in reduzierten Dosen zur Narkoseeinleitung verabreicht werden.

Die Narkose zur Sectio caesarea, häufig ultima ratio der Geburtshilfe, muß, wenn es Mutter oder Kind „schlecht geht" gleichfalls als Risikoeingriff angesehen werden. Die Einleitung und Aufrechterhaltung der Betäubung mit Methohexital bis zur vollständigen Kindesentwicklung verhindert eine weitere Depression der in vielen Fällen bereits intrauterin gefährdeten, kindlichen Vitalfunktionen.

Zusammenfassend kann festgestellt werden, daß sich das ultrakurzwirkende Oxybarbiturat Methohexital wegen seiner guten pharmakologischen Eigenschaften, seiner nur geringen Nebenwirkungen und des fast völligen Fehlens von Kontraindikationen zur Einleitung und Aufrechterhaltung der Narkose in Risikofällen besonders bewährt.

Zusammenfassung

Es werden die Bedingungen, die an ein im Rahmen der Risikoanaesthesie verwendetes Kurznarkotikum zu stellen sind, dargelegt. Diese Anforderungen erfüllt Methohexital aufgrund seines schnellen Wirkungseintritts, der kurzen Wirkungsdauer, der nur geringen Nebeneffekte auf Herz, Kreislauf, Atmung, Leber und Niere, sowie des fast völligen Fehlens kumulativer Eigenschaften weitestgehend. Seine besonderen Vorzüge bei Risikonarkosen alter Kranker, Polytraumatisierter, neurochirurgischer Patienten, Lungen-, Leber- und Nierengeschädigter, sowie bei der Sectio caesarea werden eingehend dargestellt.

Summary

The demands made on a short-acting anaesthetic in high-risk anaesthesia are discussed. Due to the rapid onset of its effect, the short duration of its action, the slightness of its side-effect on the heart, circulation, respiration, hepatic and renal functions, and its almost complete lack of any tendency to accumulate, methohexital widely complies with these requirements.

Its particular advantages in high-risk anaesthesia in the elderly, in patients with multiple injuries, in neurosurgery, pulmonary, hepatic, and renal damage, as well as in caesarian section are discussed in detail.

Literatur

1. AHNEFELD, F. W., ISRANG, H. H., HALMÁGYI, M., HEYMER, G.: Thantogenetische Faktoren bei Eingriffen im höheren Lebensalter. Anaesth. und Wiederbel. **47**, 152 (1970).
2. BELLVILLE, J. W., FENNEL, P. J., MURPHY, T., HOWLAND, W. S.: The relative potencies of Methohexital and Thiopental. J. of Pharm. and Exp. Therap. **129**, No. 1 (1960).
3. BENKE, A.: Geriatrische Anaesthesie. Anaesth. u. Wiederbel. **47**, 108 (1970).
4. BINKERT, E.: Vergleichende Untersuchungen über die Straßenverkehrstauglichkeit nach Thiopental- und Methohexital-Kurznarkosen. Schweiz. Med. Wschr. **91**, 1285 (1961).
5. BITTRICH, N. M., KANE, A. V., MOSHER, R. E.: Methohexital and its effect on liver function tests. Anesthesiology **24**, 81 (1963).
6. CLERGET, O., COUINAUD, C.: Utilisation en chirurgie générale du Méthohexital à propos de 250 observations. Anesth. Analg. Réanimation **22**, No 2 (1965).
7. COLEMAN, D. J., VILLIERS, J. C.: Anaesthesia and stereotactic surgery. Anaesthesia **19**, 60 (1964).
8. CRANDELL, D. L., WINSTON-SALEM, N. C.: The Anesthetic Hazards in Patients on Antihypertensive Therapy. J.A.M.A. **179**, No 7 (1962).
9. COLEMAN, J., GREEN, R. A.: Methohexital – a short acting barbiturate. Anaesthesia **15**, No 4 (1960).
10. DUNDEE, J. W., MOORE, J.: Thiopentone and Methohexital. Anaesthesia **16**, No 1 (1961).
11. — — The effect of scopolamine on Methohexital anaesthesia. Anaesthesia **16**, No 2 (1961).

12. Dundee, J. W., Riding, J. E., Barron, D. W., Nicholl, R. M.: Some Factors Influencing The Induction Characteristics of Methohexitone Anaesthesia. Brit. J. Anaesth. 33, 296 (1961).
13. — Moore, J.: The Effects of Premedication with Phenothiazine Derivatives on the Course of Methohexitone Anaesthesia. Brit. J. Anaesth. 33, 382 (1961).
14. — Clinical Studies of Induction Agents. Brit. J. Anaesth. 35, 784 (1963).
15. — Charakteristika bei intravenöser Narkoseeinleitung. Anaesthesist 11, 272 (1962).
16. Elliot, C. J. R., Green, R., Howells, T. H., Long, H. A.: Recovery after intravenous barbiturate Anaesthesia.
17. Gersmeyer, E. F., Yasargil, E. C.: Schock- und Kollapsfibel. Thieme Verlag 1970.
18. Hargrove, R. L., Pearce, D. J.: An anaesthetic technique for bronchoskopy. Anaesthesia 19, 226 (1964).
19. Hudson, M. W. P.: Methohexitone. The Practioner 194, 421 (1965).
20. Hügin, W.: Fragen der Anaesthesie bei Patienten, die unter Hochdruckbehandlung stehen. Anaesthesist 12, 280 (1963).
21. Hutschenreuter, K.: Anaesthesie und Notfallmedizin. Anaesth. und Wiederbel. 15, Springer-Verlag 1966.
22. Jolly, C.: Recovery time from Methohexital Anaesthesia. Brit. J. Anaesth. 32, 576 (1960).
23. Landauer, B. G.: Narkose bei Polytraumatisierten. Vortrag anläßlich des 3. Europ. Anaesthesiekongresses 1970 in Prag.
24. Lawin, P.: Alter Patient und Anaesthesie. Anaesthesist 14, 103 (1965).
25. Lehmann, Ch., Elgert, K. Weber, K.: Klinische Erfahrungen mit Methohexital-Kurznarkosen. Z. prakt. Anästh. 1, 387 (1966).
26. Simpson, R. E.: Safety and efficiency of methohexital in dental office Anaesthesia. J. canad. Dent. Ass. 32, 21 (1966).
27. Schaudig, H.: Anaesthesie im höheren Lebensalter aus chirurgischer Sicht. Anaesth. u. Wiederbel. 47, 123 (1970).
28. Thornton, H. L., Knight, P. F.: Emergency Anaesthesia. Arnold/London 1965.
29. Weinstock, S. S.: Methohexital Sodium Anaesthesia for the ambulant dental Patient. O. S., O. M. and O. P. 13, 1075 (1960).
30. Welles, J. S., McMahon, R. E., Doran, W. J.: The Metabolism and Excretion of Methohexital in rat and dog. J. of pharm. and exper. Therapeutics 139, 166 (1963).
31. Wiemers, K.: Postoperative Frühkomplikationen. Thieme Verlag 1969.

Brietal Sodium in Children's Surgery

By **B. Kay**

Derbyshire Childrens Hospital, Derby, England

You have already heard from previous speakers details of the pharmacology of methohexitone, and its use as an intravenous induction agent. I will speak mainly about the use of methohexitone in children's surgery.

In the Derbyshire Hospital for Sick Children in Derby, methohexitone is currently used to induce anaesthesia in over 90% of all cases. This is not because it is a laid-down regime, or because other induction agents are not freely available. This situation has developed spontaneously because methohexitone is the best drug in our circumstances, and has given generally better results in our hands.

Up to ten years ago the majority of children undergoing anaesthesia in Derby were subjected to gaseous induction, but about that time, under the influence of Dr. JACKSON-REES, intravenous induction became more popular throughout the whole age range. Thiopentone was the agent most commonly used at that time, as we were all well-versed in its application. When venepuncture was difficult, especially up to about 3 years of age, thiopentone was occasionally used by rectal instillation.

After 1 or 2 years methohexitone began to replace thiopentone as the induction agent of choice. Initially, it was used selectively as the more suitable barbiturate when a short duration of action was required, or better vasomotor stability and maintenance of blood pressure were necessary. However, it soon became apparent that methohexitone was in many ways a generally better intravenous induction agent than thiopentone in our pediatric practice and the use of thiopentone dwindled away so that it is now virtually never used. In our opinion it is an obsolete drug. Let me list the main advantages of methohexitone over thiopentone:

1. It is more rapidly metabolised. Not only does this mean
a) a shorter duration of action following a normal sleep-inducing dose. but also
b) a shorter duration of unwanted side-effects on the respiratory and circulatory system.
and

c) less cumulative effect, should subsequent doses of methohexitone be required, as in the intermittent-dose techniques.
also

e) an early loss of the periods of post-anaesthetic sleepiness described by DOENICKE.

2. Methohexitone causes less fall in blood pressure than thiopentone. This is not only well-documented, but is easily observed in clinical practice.

3. It is also claimed that methohexitone causes less respiratory depression than thiopentone. In our experience this is very dependant on the method of use, but it is certain that minimum sleep doses given at the optimum rate cause minimal respiratory effects.

4. The claim that methohexitone causes a smaller incidence of laryngeal spasm than thiopentone is borne out by our experience, and is important in our practice where injection is usually followed by rapid induction by nitrous oxide, oxygen and halothane breathed spontaneously, the halothane being administered in the highest concentration the child will accept.

5. Thiopentone undoubtedly causes more tissue damage than equipotent concentrations of methohexitone if given intra-arterially, or extra-vascularly. This is of great importance in pediatric practice where it is easy to miss an intravenous injection in a small squirming child.

6. This non-irritant feature of methohexitone increases its versatility of use, and allows it to be used by intramuscular injection as well as by intravenous or rectal use like thiopentone.

7. Methohexitone solutions are much more stable than thiopentone solutions, remaining fit for use for several weeks at room temperature, resulting in convenience and economy in use.
There were two disadvantages that methohexitone suffered in comparison with thiopentone.

Firstly, there is an increased incidence of post-injection involuntary movement. This effect is very dependant on the method of administration, including pre-operative medication, thoroughly studied by DUNDEE and his colleagues. In our experience the two main causes were size and rate of dosage and by adopting our basic principles of giving minimal sleep-inducing doses at optimal slow rates of injection we virtually eliminated this problem.

Secondly, some children experienced pain in the arm during intravenous injection of methohexitone. This pain originates in the vein, but is usually experienced in the upper arm or shoulder. We experimented with different concentrations and rates of injection but found that it could only be eli-

Two further developments coincided with the elimination of thiopentone from our practice, firstly the application of our "minimal disturbance" techniques with concealed intravenous injection. This allowed even more general adoption of intravenous induction, with the least psychological disturbance of the child. I will give more details later. Secondly we began to treat the majority of children undergoing non-emergency surgery as outpatients. The adoption of this desirable practice was greatly facilitated by our established use of methohexitone.

In late 1965 propanidid became available, and we gave the drug an extensive trial for the next $2^1/_2$ years, involving about 5000 cases. Eventually the use of propanidid dwindled away, leaving methohexitone again employed as our induction agent of choice. The main reasons were these:

1. Propanidid is very viscous. It requires a big needle, and such cannot always be inserted into a young child's small veins.

2. There was an immediate increase in the incidence of post-operative vomiting, negligable with methohexitone, and very undesirable in outpatients.

3. There was also an immediate increase in the incidence of troublesome venous thromboses, again negligable with methohexitone.

4. We did not experience a reduction of post-injection involuntary movement with propanidid. The incidence remained much the same as that occurring after methohexitone as we used it.

5. There was little advantage in the shorter duration of action of propanidid in our practice. When used as an induction agent before inhalation anaesthesia the length of action becomes less important, and even though many of our patients are out-patients, being children and accompanied by parents "street-consciousness" is not of importance in the majority. Propanidid is still used for older children leaving the hospital soon after short operations, but its short action is not required in other cases. Occasionally it can be troublesome. When some trainee anaesthetists are taking a long time over establishment of inhalation anaesthesia (relaxation, laryngoscopy, local anaesthetic spray and intubation) consciousness may return too early.

6. We expected propanidid to be superior to methohexitone for intermittent intravenous anaesthetics. However, in our hands it is not so, the more sudden return of consciousness and activity making for a jerky and uneven anaesthetic progress, more difficult to manage.

7. Cardiovascular stability. Although in general there was little difference in the cardiovascular responses of our patients following induction by

children displayed an abnormal reaction to propanidid. This was characterized by an acute exanthamatous reaction covering the whole body and accompanied by gross hypotension requiring heroic resuscitation measures. A third similar case was published by a colleague, these three occurring in our series of 5000 cases. He gave reasons for believing the reaction to be an allergic phenomenon, probably with gross histamine release, and I believe DOENICKE has evidence to support this theory. Since our publication many more reports of this phenomenon have appeared including some in adults, and at least one resulting in the death of the patient. We regard the incidence of such a dangerous complication to be unacceptably high to allow us to use propanidid routinely, and now reserve it for the special circumstances outlined. During the last 6 months we have investigated the use of ketamine for anaesthesia and induction of anaesthesia. This unusual agent certainly has a place in pediatric practice, as the post-anaesthetic hallucinations are not so troublesome as in adults, and the hypertensive response generally not so dangerous. However, it is not a short-acting drug and usually not suitable as our established techniques for out-patient work, especially as post-operative vomiting is encountered much more frequently. Also the present cost would mitigate against its use simply as an induction agent, where it offers little advantage. We now use it selectively for a few special procedures, for instance operations in the mouth, antral wash-out etc.

I have explained the development of our methods of induction of anaesthesia for children at some length because we believe that the experience is of enormous importance to any child unfortunate enough to have to undergo it. Induction must inevitably place a stress on the child, and we have for some years investigated the important causes of this stress, and the ways of reducing it to a minimum.

We measured the child's distress in 2 ways, first by observation of the child's behaviour in the anaesthetic room, at different stages of preparation and induction, rating the distress from 1–5. A second evaluation was made by questionaire comparing the child's behaviour at home before and after operation. The 2 methods produced closely parallel results.

The method of induction of anaesthesia was found to be important and produced clear-cut results. There is no doubt at all that our method of inducing sleep by a concealed painless intravenous injection causes significantly less disturbance to the child during induction when compared with ordinary intravenous injection or nitrous oxide, oxygen and halothane induction even by an expert. This is even more clearly seen in the second method of assessment.

Another method of clearly reducing distress was to allow the mother to

most consistantly by concealed painless intravenous injection of methohexitone.

Our general approach based on minimal distress for the child undergoing out-patient surgery is therefore as follows:

1. Mother present whenever the child is conscious (during induction and recovery).

2. No premedication or other preoperative injection. A technique has been developed to reduce pre-operative apprehension without the use of sedatives, including an earlier visit to the anaesthetic room to meet the anaesthetist and play with the toys there.

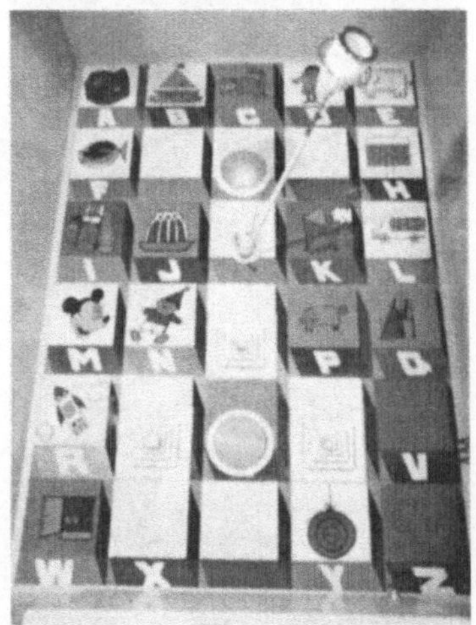

Fig. 1. The ceiling of the anaesthetic room

3. Little disturbance of the childs clothing. Many children resent intrusions on their privacy, and undressing is done after they are asleep.

4. Continuation of play or entertainment and the provision of an anaesthetic room suitable for an active, accompanied child. We employ an attendant who introduces the toys etc. and diverts the childs attention from his operation.

5. Concealed intravenous induction of anaesthesia.

6. Minimal restriction of food, drink or activity, particularly postoperatively.

Fig. 1. shows the ceiling of our anaesthetic room, not so often seen as many inductions take place with the child on the mother's knee (Fig. 2).

The slide shows how the attendant constricts the wrist to prevent venous return, and at the same time obstructs the childs view of the injection site. This is then sprayed from 5–8 sec with ethyl chloride, *not* to the point of freezing of tissues, and the injection can be made without any sensation. The ethyl chloride spray has previously been introduced to the child in play as a "cold-water pistol", and if the child is too interested a spectator a diversionary spraying of the other, visible hand is carried out whilst the injection is made.

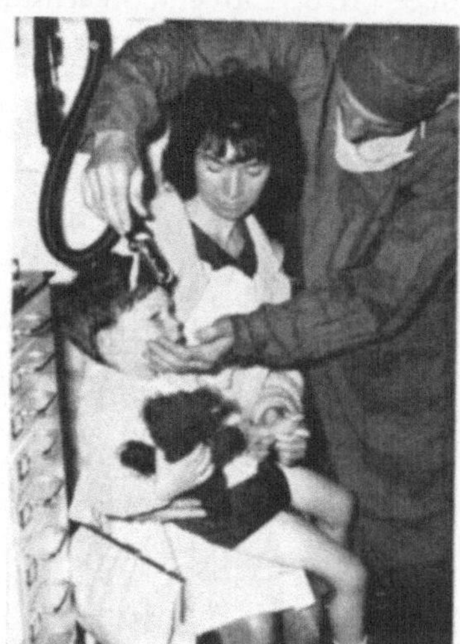

Fig. 2. Induction of anaesthesia with the child on the mother's knee

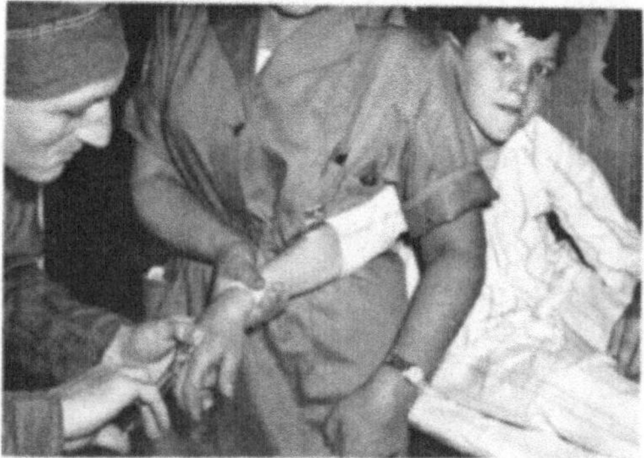

Fig. 3. The "concealed" intravenous induction

We use 1% methohexitone, injected slowly until the desired depth of sleep is achieved. We use relatively small doses to produce light sleep with no respiratory depression so that uptake of inhalation agents is rapid. Our usual dose-level is between 1.0 and 1.5 mg/kg or approximately 0.5 ml per year of age.

The problem of venous pain was solved by adding a small amount of lignocaine to this solution – 1 ml of 1% lignocaine in 10 mls 1% methohexitone is safe and suitable, but we usually draw a few drops of 2% lignocaine into our syringe containing a smaller dose. A small precipitate occurs, that disappears on shaking. We also add atropine (omitted pre-operatively) to our methohexitone if it is desired.

This remains our standard induction method whenever intravenous injection is feasible. It is most difficult between the ages of 6 months and 18 months in our population, and in these children rectal methohexitone is frequently used in a dose of 5 mg/kg, given as a 5% solution. This usually produces light, transient sleep in about 10 min, and the dose can be doubled if true basal narcosis is required.

Intramuscular methohexitone is popular with a number of pediatric anaesthetists, and is very effective especially in children up to about 8 years old. A dose of 4 mg/kg in 2% solution is effective in producing light sleep in about 5 min, but more can be given for deeper hypnosis. However, the injection is painful, especially with the larger volumes required for older children, and it does not fit in with our attempts at painless induction.

I have spoken largely about the induction of sleep before inhalation anaesthesia, our general use of methohexitone. Obviously, however, it is frequently used as the sole agent for short procedures, such as incision of abscess or reduction of a fracture. In this role it is superior to thiopentone and about as efficient as propanidid. We prefer it in children for the reasons already given.

Methohexitone is also the most suitable agent for intermittent intravenous anaesthesia, for producing very light prolonged sleep to cover an unpleasant procedure involving little pain. This is important to note, as methohexitone has little analgesic effectiveness and attempts to prevent reflex movements to painful stimuli result in an unwanted depth of anaesthesia with respiratory depression and lack of airway control. These problems have been noted in publications criticizing the method, whilst attempting to employ it in unsuitable circumstances or for unsuitable procedures.

We have used the intermittent Brietal technique extensively to provide ultra-light anaesthesia for children undergoing such procedures as extensive dental conservation and myelography. Here deeper anaesthesia can

to severe stimulation. In dental work this technique can also be modified
by using the ultra light sleep in conjunction with an intravenously administered analgesic (we use pentazocine) instead of local anaesthetic
block. Obviously much-reduced doses of methohexitone are required.

I have explained to you our reasons for preferring methohexitone in
pediatric anaesthesia, and our methods of using it. Both have now stood
the test of time and even after eight years there seems to be no alternative
product which is so generally useful, or so safe.

Summary

In Derbyshire Hospital for Sick Children in Derby, methohexital is
employed in 96% of all inductions of anaesthesia. Induction via inhalation,
formely exercised, is omitted virtually on principle.

Thiopental, which was used in the interim, is regarded as obsolete, since
methohexital shows a shorter duration of action, its side effects on the respiratory and circulatory systems subside more rapidly, and its cumulative
effect is modest. Moreover, the postanaesthetic somnolence it causes re-
solves within a shorter period of time. Furthermore, the fall in the blood
pressure following methohexital is less pronounced. This anaesthetic rarely
causes laryngospasm and leads to no more than slight tissural damage on
extravascular injection. Owing to this latter property, methohexital may be
given intramuscularly and per rectum. Solutions of methohexital are most
stable and may be used for several weeks when kept at room temperature.

The observed disadvantages of this anaesthetic consist in a higher incidence of involuntary movements, as well as pain irradiating from the site of
injection to the body.

Propanidide did not prove satisfactory, since its injection requires large-
bore cannulas. Moreover, it produces postoperative vomiting and venous
thrombosis and is not suitable for intermittent administration. Additionally,
a severe drop in the blood pressure was occasionally observed which required heroic resuscitation procedures, accompanied by the development
of acute eczema. These symptoms must be regarded as manifestations of
excessive release of histamine.

Ketanest which has likewise held its ground in paediatric practice, since
the postanaesthetic hallucinations and the hypertonic reactions are not so
hazardous and disagreeable, is not a short-acting preparation and is, therefore, not suitable for out-patient treatment. We have frequently observed
administration of this preparation to cause vomitting and have, therefore,
restricted its use to special cases.

ethylene chloride onto the site of puncturing. Then he performs the injection without the child being able to watch the procedure.

Venous pain is excluded by adding small amounts of lidocaine to the methohexital solution (1 ml of a 1% solution of lidocaine to 10 ml of a 1% solution of methohexital). Any slight precipitation occurring in the mixture is readily removed by shaking the syringe. Likewise, the injection solution contains atropine, since pretreatment per se is omitted.

For rectal application, 5 mg/kg are given as a 5% solution, for intramuscular injection, 4 mg/kg as a 2% solution.

Zusammenfassung

Das Derbyshire Hospital für kranke Kinder in Derby verwendet in 90% aller Narkoseeinleitungen Methohexital, verzichtet jetzt also fast grundsätzlich auf die früher durchgeführte Inhalationseinleitung.

Thiopental, das zwischenzeitlich genommen wurde, wird als veraltet betrachtet, weil Methohexital eine kürzere Wirkungsdauer, eine kürzere Dauer unerwünschter Nebenwirkungen auf das Atmungs- und Kreislaufsystem, einen geringeren kumulativen Effekt und einen frühzeitigen Schwund postanästhetischer Schläfrigkeitsperioden aufweist. Methohexital bewirkt weiterhin geringeren Blutdruckabfall, selteneres Auftreten eines Laryngospasmus und unbeträchtlichere Gewebsschäden bei extravasaler Verabreichung. Diese letzte Eigenschaft gestattet sowohl eine intramuskuläre Injektion als auch eine rektale Applikation.

Methohexitallösungen sind stabiler und bleiben bei Zimmertemperatur etliche Wochen lang gebrauchsfähig.

Die beobachteten Nachteile sind eine vermehrte Häufigkeit unwillkürlicher Bewegungen und von der Injektionsstelle körperwärts ziehende Schmerzen.

Propanidid bewährte sich nicht, weil es wegen seiner Viskosität große Injektionsnadeln erfordert, postoperatives Erbrechen verursacht, Venenthrombosen auslöst und zur intermittierenden Verabreichung nicht verwendet werden kann. Wir sahen zusätzlich starke Blutdruckabfälle, die heroische Wiederbelebungsmaßnahmen erforderten und von akuten Exanthemen begleitet wurden. Diese Symptome müssen als Ausdruck exzessiver Histaminfreisetzung gewertet werden.

Ketanest, dem sein Platz in der pädiatrischen Praxis nicht abgesprochen werden kann, weil die postnarkotischen Halluzinationen und die hypertonen Reaktionen hier nicht so unangenehm und gefährlich sind, ist kein kurz-

Die Angst des Kindes vor der intravenösen Injektion wird durch die „verborgene" Einleitung ausgeschlossen. Der Anaesthesist komprimiert das Handgelenk, staut also die Venen, sprüht 5 bis 8 Sekunden lang Chloräthyl auf die Einstichstelle und injiziert, ohne daß das Kind den Vorgang beobachten kann.

Der Venenschmerz wird durch den Zusatz kleiner Mengen von Lidocain zur Methohexitallösung (1 ml 1%iges Lidocain in 10 ml 1%igem Methohexital) vermieden. Geringfügige Ausfälle werden durch Schütteln der Spritze beseitigt. Die gleiche Lösung enthält Atropin, weil von einer eigentlichen Prämedikation abgesehen wird.

Bei der rektalen Anwendung werden 5 mg/kg als 5%ige Lösung, bei der intramuskulären 4 mg/kg als 2%ige Lösung gegeben.

Kombinationsnarkose mit Methohexital bei Risikopatienten in der Urologie

Von **K. Weber** und **G. Gross**

Aus der Anaesthesie-Abteilung
des St. Elisabeth-Krankenhauses Köln-Hohenlind
(Chefarzt: Dr. K. Weber)

Wir haben die Wirksamkeit von Methohexital an 365 Patienten untersucht, die sich einem endovesikalen Eingriff unterziehen mußten.

Die Altersverteilung unseres Krankengutes ersehen Sie aus Abbildung 1.

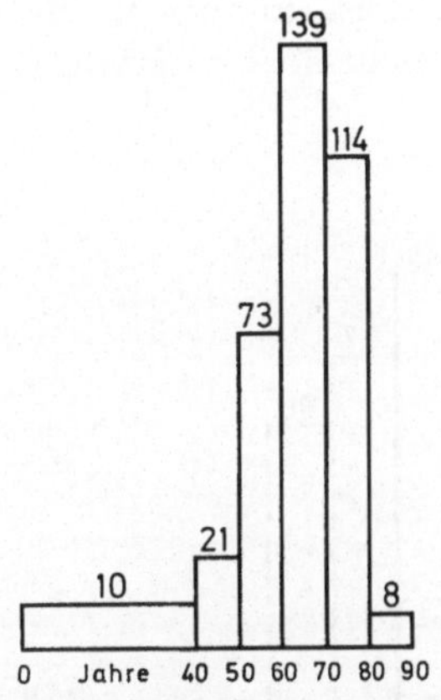

Abb. 1. Altersverteilung des Krankengutes

Hierbei wird ohne weiteres deutlich, daß 261 Patienten, das sind mehr als 70%, in die Gruppe des 7.–9. Lebensjahrzehntes fallen.

Zur Erläuterung ist weiterhin anzumerken, daß es sich nicht um ausgewählte Fälle, sondern um das routinemäßige Krankengut einer urologischen Abteilung handelt.

218 Patienten, das sind 60%, waren an einem Prostataadenom erkrankt.

wurden und bei der 6. vorwiegend um Vasotomien handelt, die meistens gleichzeitig mit dem endovesicalen Eingriff vorgenommen wurden.

Tabelle 1. *Zusammenfassung der Diagnosen*

	Fälle
Prostataadenom	218
Blasenpapillom	39
Sonst. Blasen- u. Harnr.Erkr.	37
Harnleiterstein	29
Blasencarcinom	19
Orchitis u. Epididymitis	13
Prostatacarcinom	10

Die weitere Charakteristik unseres Krankengutes ist dem hohen Alter der Patienten entsprechend gekennzeichnet durch die große Zahl interner Begleiterkrankungen, wie Lungenemphysem, pathologische EKG-Werte, Hypertonie, Diabetes mellitus, chronische Bronchitis usw. (Abb. 2). Die Abbildung gibt eine Übersicht über die häufigsten Alterskrankheiten überhaupt.

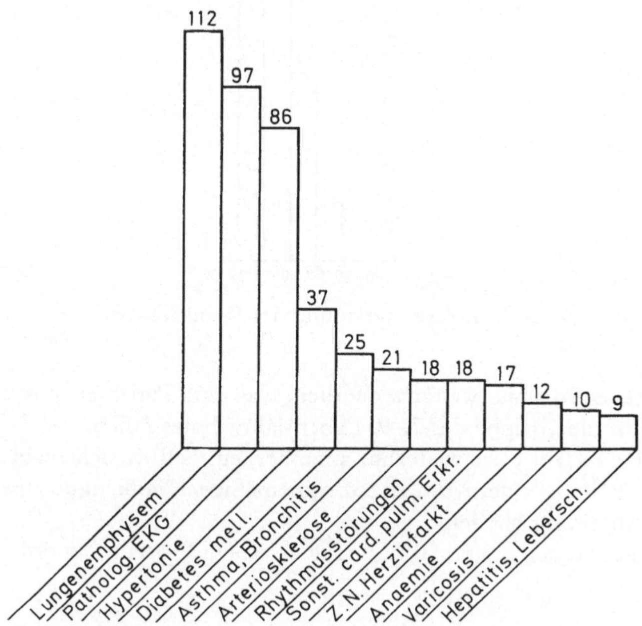

Abb. 2. Übersicht über die internen Begleiterkrankungen

Diese Begleiterkrankungen waren den Patienten teilweise schon sehr lange bekannt, teilweise wurden sie erst bei der Operations- und Narkosevorbereitung aufgedeckt.

Die Kriterien für die dargestellten Diagnosen waren klinische Untersuchung, Röntgenaufnahme der Lunge, Elektrokardiogramm und Laboratoriumsbefunde. Hypertonie bestand bei Blutdruckwerten von über 160 mmHg systolisch, Diabetes bei Nüchternblutzuckerwerten von über 150 mg% nach einer enzymatischen Methode.

Unter der Rubrik „sonstige kardiopulmonale Begleiterkrankungen" wurden eine früher durchgemachte Lungenembolie oder Tuberkulose, mit Hilfe von Strophanthin oder Digitalis präoperativ kompensierte, vorher manifeste Rechts- oder Linksherzinsuffizienz oder ein Cor pulmonale zusammengefaßt.

Die Prämedikation bestand in Applikation von durchschnittlich 2 ml Thalamonal und 0,5 mg Atropin intramuskulär eine halbe Stunde vor Beginn der Anaesthesie.

Im Operationssaal wurde nach Blutdruckmessung und Anlage einer intravenösen Verweilkanüle zunächst mit einer Infusion von 5%iger Glukoselösung, bei Diabetes oder Leberschädigung mit Laevulose – oder 10%iger Xylit-Lösung begonnen. Unmittelbar danach erfolgte die Injektion von 80–120 mg Methohexital in 1%iger Lösung.

Die Narkose wurde fortgesetzt mit einem Sauerstoff-Lachgas-Gemisch im Verhältnis 1:2 – bei einem Flow von 6 l/min – unter assistierender Maskenbeatmung im halbgeschlossenen Kreissystem.

In den meisten Fällen wurde Halothan in einer Konzentration von 0,3–0,5 Vol.% zugegeben. Hierbei ist zu bemerken, daß wir bei diesem niedrigen Halothanzusatz depressive Nebenwirkungen auf das Herz und Gefäßsystem – selbst bei cardial erheblich vorgeschädigten Patienten – nicht beobachteten.

5 min nach dem Beginn mit Methohexital injizierten wir 2 ml Thalamonal intravenös. Dieser 5 minütige Abstand zwischen der Methohexital- und der Thalamonalinjektion wurde aus verschiedenen Gründen eingehalten: es gelingt hiermit, bereits in den Wirkungsabfall des Methohexital hinein zu injizieren, vielleicht sogar die Wirkung von Methohexital zu potenzieren und zu verlängern.

Eine sofortige Injektion von Thalamonal (sofort nach Methohexital) würde infolge des gefäßerweiternden Effektes des Dehydrobenzperidolanteils zu einem unerwünschten Blutdruckabfall führen, zumal zu diesem Zeitpunkt noch nicht genügend Infusionsflüssigkeit zum prophylaktischen Volumenausgleich dieser Gefäßerweiterung eingelaufen ist.

Zur besseren Ruhigstellung des Operationsgebietes, auch zur Erleichterung der Beatmung waren zuweilen fraktionierte Dosen von Succinylcholin erforderlich (Tab. 2).

Tabelle 2. *Prämedikation nnd Narkose*

Prämedikation	2 ml Thalamonal 0,5 mg Atropin
Narkose	1. Anlage einer Infusion von 500 ml 5 %iger Glucose oder Laevulose 2. Methohexital 80–120 mg i. v. 3. $O_2 : N_2O = 2:4$ l/min, Halothan 0,3–0,7 vol % mit assistierter Maskenbeatmung 4. Thalamonal 2 ml, 5 min nach Methohexital 5. Relaxierung mit Succinyl nach Bedarf

Auf die Intubation konnte in den meisten Fällen verzichtet werden.

Die Narkose wurde beendet unter allmählicher Rückkehr der Spontanatmung bei Gabe von reinem Sauerstoff.

Mit der angegebenen Narkosetechnik schlafen die Patienten störungsfrei und rasch ein, sind ausreichend analgesiert und postoperativ weitgehend ruhiggestellt, jedoch sofort wieder im vollständigen Besitz aller Vitalfunktionen.

Am Operationstag geben wir insgesamt 2 l Flüssigkeit intravenös, die sich aus Glucose, Laevulose und Vollelektrolytlösung zusammensetzt. Blutverluste werden zusätzlich mit Dextran, bei Bedarf durch Bluttransfusionen ausgeglichen. Am Abend des Operationstages können die Patienten nach Belieben trinken.

Die Dauer der Anaesthesie kann sich, für den Anaesthesisten und den Operateur vorher meist nicht bestimmbar, bis über 2 Std erstrecken. Bei 70%, also 256 Patienten, betrug sie bis zu einer Std (Tabelle 3).

Tabelle 3. *Dauer der Narkose*

		Fälle
bis	30 min	108
bis	60 min	148
bis	90 min	77
bis	120 min	26
über	120 min	6

Tabelle 4. *Kreislaufverhalten während der Narkose*

Abfall		Anstieg
181	0–10	62
53	10–20	26
13	20–30	11
12	30–40	3
4	40–50	—
Fälle	mmHg	Fälle

Hier ist ersichtlich, daß es in den weitaus überwiegenden Fällen, nämlich 243, lediglich zu Schwankungen von plus/minus 10 mmHg systolisch kam.

Zugrundegelegt wurden nur die Blutdruckwerte innerhalb der ersten 15 min nach Beginn der Narkose, da für spätere Blutdruckänderungen nicht die Kombination von Methohexital und Thalamonal, sondern vielmehr Blutverlust im Operationsgebiet und dessen nicht zeitgerechter Ersatz verantwortlich zu machen sein dürfte (Abb. 3).

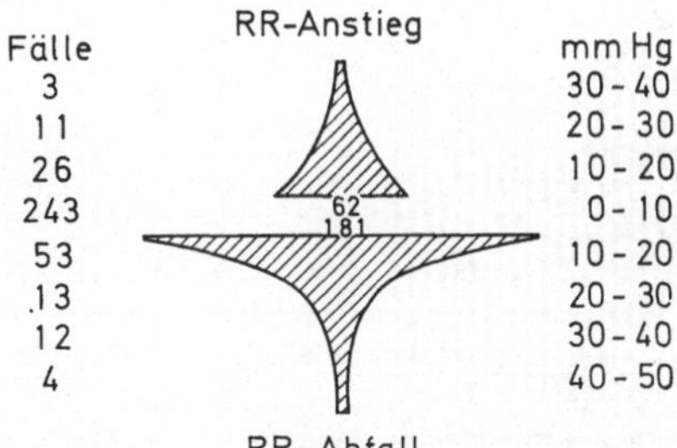

Abb. 3. Kreislaufverhalten während der Narkose

Aus dieser Darstellung wird besonders deutlich, daß insgesamt 322 Fälle Blutdruckschwankungen von plus/minus 20 mmHg systolisch aufweisen, das sind 88%, während nur 43, das sind 12%, größere Blutdruck-Abfälle oder -Anstiege zeigten, welche nur in Einzelfällen über 40 mmHg hinausgingen.

In Relation zu den schweren Begleiterkrankungen unserer Patienten – allein 86, das sind etwa 24%, litten an einer Hypertonie, welche teilweise mit Ganglioplegica anbehandelt worden war – ergibt sich gerade in dieser Kreislaufstabilität eine wichtige Eigenschaft der angewandten Kombinationsnarkose.

Zur weiteren Verdeutlichung dürfen wir den Narkoseverlauf eines 83jährigen Patienten zeigen, bei dem die Elektroresektion eines Prostataadenoms vorgenommen wurde. Der Patient hatte eine Hypertonie, ein Lungenemphysem mit Cor pulmonale und vor 2 Jahren einen elektro-kardiographisch und klinisch nachgewiesenen Herzinfarkt durchgemacht. Sie sehen völlig stabile Blutdruckverhältnisse nach typischer Methohexital-Thalamonal-Injektion (Abb. 4).

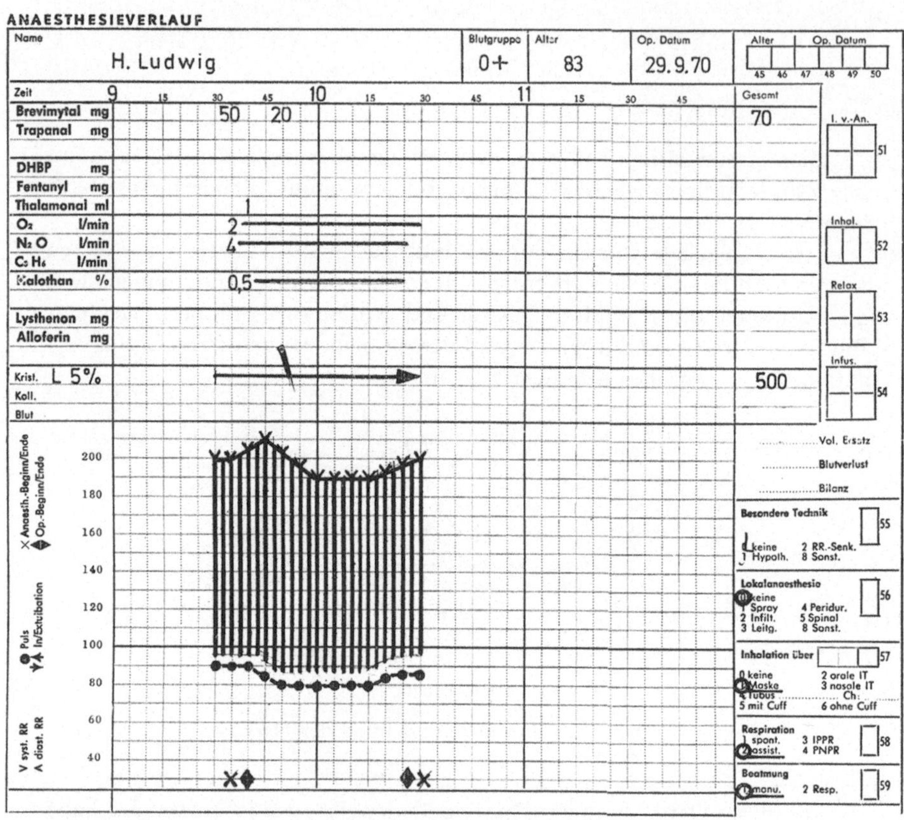

Abb. 4. Narkoseverlauf bei einem 83jährigen Patienten mit Hypertonie, Lungen-emphysem mit Cor pulmonale und nach einem 2 Jahre vorher durchgemachten Herzinfarkt (Elektroresektion eines Prostataadenoms)

In Abbildung 5 ist der Narkoseverlauf bei einem 81jährigen Patienten wiedergegeben, bei dem ebenfalls die Elektroresektion eines Prostata-adenoms durchgeführt wurde. Bei diesem Patienten haben wir präoperativ eine Rechtsherzinsuffizienz mit arterieller Hypertonie, Lungenemphysem und asthmatoider Bronchitis festgestellt. Auch hier ist ein glatter, stabiler Narkoseverlauf zu beobachten.

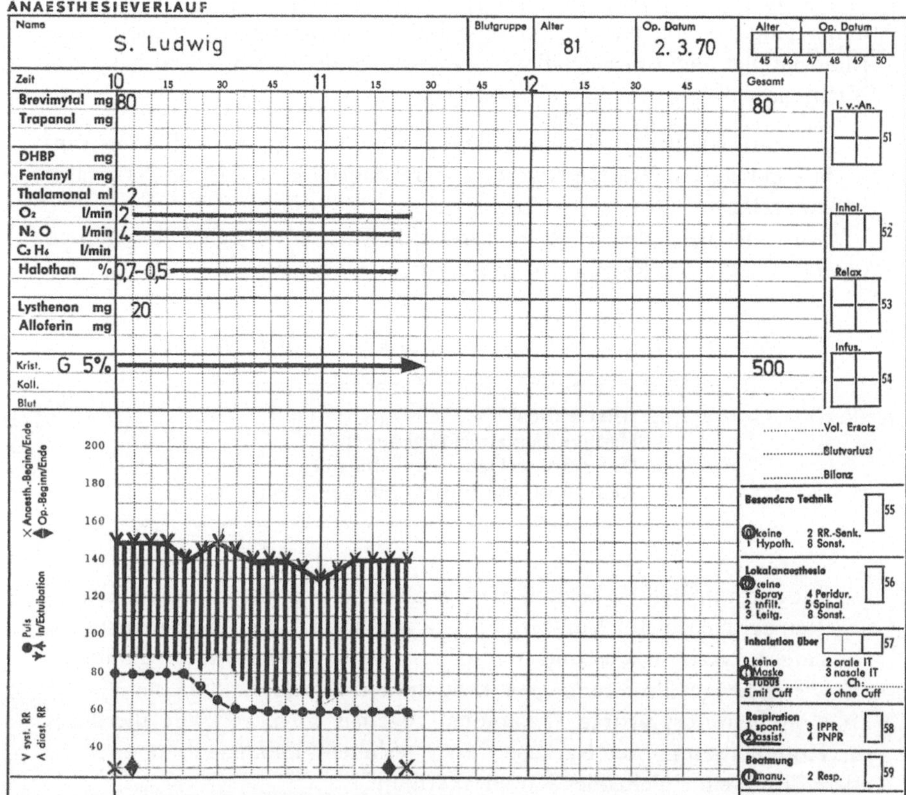

Abb. 5. Narkoseverlauf bei einem 81jährigen Patienten, bei dem präoperativ eine
Rechtsinsuffizienz mit arterieller Hypertonie, Lungenemphysem und asthmatoider
Bronchitis festgestellt wurde (Elektroresektion eines Prostataadenoms)

Bei der Diskussion der angewandten Anaesthesietechnik ist auf die
besonderen Charakteristiken einer Narkose bei endovesicalen Eingriffen
hinzuweisen. Diese Charakteristiken sind bereits aus dem vorher Gesagten
deutlich geworden. Alter und gravierende Begleiterkrankungen ergeben
ein hohes Narkoserisiko (Tab. 5).

Aus diesen Gründen wird auch heute noch einer Spinal- oder Peri-
dural-Anaesthesie mancherorts der Vorzug gegeben.

Das Risiko einer Allgemeinnarkose wurde jedoch durch die Entwicklung moderner Pharmaka, welche die einzelnen Qualitäten der Narkose
besser steuerbar machten, bedeutend herabgesetzt. Die Mononarkose alten
Stils wurde abgelöst durch eine Kombinationsanaesthesie, die es erlaubt,
differente Eigenschaften einzelner Pharmaka zielgerecht auszunutzen.

Die heutige Neuroleptanalgesie (NLA) stellt den vorläufigen Abschluß dieser Entwicklung dar. Im Spezialgebiet der endovesicalen urologischen Eingriffe hat die routinemäßige Anwendung der NLA allerdings zwei Nachteile:

1. kann, wie bereits erwähnt, die Operationsdauer vor Beginn des Eingriffs nicht genau festgelegt werden, der Eingriff kann für die NLA also zu kurz sein,

2. ist die bei jeder NLA zu fordernde Intubation bei endovesicalen Operationen in der Regel nicht notwendig.

Tabelle 5. *Charakteristik der Narkose bei endovesicalen Eingriffen*

1. Alter Patient
2. Häufige Begleiterkrankungen
3. Unbekannte Dauer des Eingriffes
4. Keine absolute Intubationsindikation

Mit der mitgeteilten Technik dagegen können wir die günstigen Eigenschaften der Neuroleptica und Analgetica ausnützen, ohne ihre ungünstigen, wie längere Narkosedauer und Atemdepression, in Kauf nehmen zu müssen.

Die niedrige Dosierung von Dehydrobenzperidol und Fentanyl, das als Kombinationspräparat Thalamonal gegeben wird, verlangt allerdings die Komplettierung der Narkose durch geringen Halothanzusatz und vor allem durch ein einleitendes Kurznarkotikum.

Hierbei hat sich uns Methohexital bereits im Zeitraum von 1961–1965 in über 10000 Fällen, worüber an anderer Stelle berichtet wurde, bewährt. Inzwischen wurden zahlreiche weitere Erfahrungen gesammelt.

Seit Mai 1969 haben wir in mindestens 6000 Fällen Methohexital als Einleitungsnarkotikum angewandt. Aus der Fülle der Vorzüge dieses Präparates, über die meine Vorredner schon berichteten, erscheinen uns immer wieder besonders bemerkenswert: die gute Venenverträglichkeit, die relativ geringen Nebenwirkungen auf Atemzentrum, Herz und Gefäß-System und die geringe Nachschlafdauer als Folge des schnellen Abbaus innerhalb des physikalischen und chemischen Wirkungsmechanismus.

Zusammenfassung

Wie unsere Darlegungen zeigten, fanden wir diese Vorzüge von Methohexital auch an unserem urologischen Krankengut in jeder Weise bestätigt. Gerade in der zeitgerechten Kombination von Methohexital mit Thalamonal, Halothan und Lachgas glauben wir eine praktikable und sichere Methode für die dargestellten Risikonarkosen gefunden zu haben.

Summary

As has been shown in this paper, we have found the advantages of methohexital to apply in all respects to our urologic patient material. Particularly in the timely combination of methohexital with Thalamonal, Halothane, and nitrous oxide we believe to have found a practicable and safe method for high-risk anaesthesia in all the conditions mentioned.

Methohexital und Kaiserschnitt

Von **H. Bauer-Ehnes**

Aus der Anaesthesie-Abteilung (Chefarzt: Dr. CH. LEHMANN)
der Chirurg. Klinik und Poliklinik (Direktor: Prof. Dr. G. MAURER)
am Klinikum rechts der Isar der Technischen Universität München

Schon die Vielzahl der für die Sectio caesarea vorgeschlagenen Anaesthesieverfahren beweist, daß es für diesen geburtshilflichen Eingriff bisher keine ideale Narkosemethode gibt.

Nach CRAWFORD sind allgemeine Kriterien, die jede geburtshilfliche Anaesthesie erfüllen sollte, völlige Schmerzausschaltung, ausreichende Sauerstoffversorgung, die Anwendung gering toxischer Medikamente, das Vermeiden von Hypotension und Erbrechen für die Mutter, die Umgehung mangelnder Sauerstoffversorgung und die Garantie minimaler zentraler Depression durch Anaesthesiemittel und Analgetica für das Kind und gute Arbeitsbedingungen für den Geburtshelfer [3].

Einige Vorbemerkungen zur Physiologie der Placenta, des Feten und der Schwangeren sollen die Problematik veranschaulichen.

Im Zentrum des Interesses steht die Durchlässigkeit der Placenta für Pharmaka. Sie ist der Durchlässigkeit der Blut-Hirn-Schranke vergleichbar und nach MOYA von Konzentrationsgradient, Diffusionsgefälle, Jonisationsgrad, Lipoidlöslichkeit und Molekulargewicht abhängig [15].

Stoffe mit einem Molekulargewicht unter 350 durchschreiten die Placenta rasch. Hierzu gehören alle Barbiturate und die meisten Analgetica. Stoffe mit einem Molekulargewicht zwischen 350 und 600, also zum Beispiel Succinylcholin, gelangen nur zögernd und in höheren Konzentrationen durch die Placentar-Schranke [15]. (MOYA u. KVISSELGARD konnten Succinylcholin erst nach der ungebräuchlich hohen, einmaligen Dosis von 300 bis 400 mg in meßbaren Mengen im Placentar-Blut nachweisen [16]). Stoffe mit einem Molekulargewicht zwischen 600 und 1000 wie Curare passieren die Placenta äußerst langsam. Für Substanzen mit einem Molekulargewicht über 1000 ist dieses Organ nahezu inpermeabel [11, 15].

Barbiturate und Analgetika besitzen außer dem niedrigen Molekulargewicht eine hohe Lipoidlöslichkeit und einen niedrigen Jonisationsgrad. Da sie eine Speicherung in Leber und Gehirn der Feten erfahren [19], stellen gefundene Nabelschnurkonzentrationen keine repräsentativen Daten dar.

Einer besonderen Beachtung bedarf die Anatomie des Ungeborenen. CRAWFORD betont, daß ein beträchtlicher Teil des von der Placenta zum Feten fließenden Blutes die Leber primär umgeht und via untere Hohlvene, rechter Vorhof, linker Vorhof, linke Kammer in die Aorta fließt [3]. Somit erhält das fetale Gehirn einen beträchtlichen Anteil der die Placenta passierenden Pharmaca, ehe sie ein anderes Kapillargebiet durchströmt haben.

Das unreife Gehirn des Ungeborenen und jungen Neugeborenen leidet laut ROTH u. BARLOW im Gegensatz zum Erwachsenen an einem Myelinmangel, der die Aufnahme auch schwer lipoidlöslicher Substanzen begünstigt [20].

Außerdem ist nach Mitteilungen von JONDORF, FONTS u. Mitarb. das Fermentsystem beim Feten bis über die Geburt hinaus mangelhaft entwickelt [5, 9]. Nach der Entbindung können metabolische Fehlleistungen für das Kind noch bedrohlichere Ausmaße annehmen, weil die Ausscheidung von Medikamenten oder ihren Metaboliten über die Placenta nicht mehr möglich ist.

JAMES nahm vergleichende Untersuchungen von vaginal- und schnittentbundenen Neugeborenen vor, deren Mütter identische Barbituratdosen erhalten hatten. Die stärkere Depression der durch Sectio caesarea geborenen Kinder erklärt er durch die ungestörte Perfusion der intervillösen Räume bei fehlender Wehentätigkeit, also aufgehobener Uteruskontraktion [8].

Die kontrollierte Beatmung der Schwangeren erfordert besondere Aufmerksamkeit und große klinische Erfahrung. Das Atemminutenvolumen der Mutter steigt im Laufe der Gravidität um ca. 42% an. Die erhöhte alveoläre Ventilation bedingt vor allem bei der Anwendung von Inhalationsanaesthetica mit hoher Blutlöslichkeit eine beschleunigte Narkose-Einleitung und ein schnelleres Abklingen der Anaesthesie [2, 4, 18].

Eine Hypoventilation führt schneller zur Hypoxie als bei Nichtschwangeren. MORISHIMA, MOYA, MOTOYAMA u. Mitarb. stellten in tierexperimentellen und klinischen Studien fest, daß eine Hyperventilation der Mutter zur Vasokonstriktion der Placentargefäße mit Gas- und Stoffwechselaustauschstörungen führen und somit ebenfalls eine fetale Hypoxie bedingen kann [13, 14, 17].

Weiterhin wird der venöse Rückstrom zum Herzen bei forcierter Überdruckbeatmung vermindert. Die dadurch abnehmende Auswurfleistung führt ihrerseits ebenfalls zur Uterusmangeldurchblutung.

Eine wesentliche Bedeutung hat das von HOLMES u. HOWARD beschriebene Vena cava-Kompressions- oder Supine-hypotensive-Syndrom [6, 7]. Im letzten Schwangerschaftsdrittel kann der Druck des Uterus bei Rückenlagerung auf die Vena cava inferior zu einem schweren, lebensbedrohlichen Schock mit Blutdruckabfall, Tachycardie und Bewußtlosigkeit führen. Bei Seitenlagerung erholt sich die Schwangere in wenigen Minuten.

Die mitgeteilten Imponderabilien bestimmen viele Anaesthesiologen, die Lokal- bzw. Leitungsanaesthesie für die geplante Schnittentbindung zu bevorzugen.

Sie hat für das Neugeborene den unbestrittenen Vorteil der fehlenden Betäubung und vermeidet eine Aspiration, die für die Mutter die Hauptgefahr der Allgemein-Anaesthesie darstellt.

Andererseits können schnell resorbierte, größere Mengen der Lokal-Anaesthetika zu Hypotonie, Schock und Irritation des Zentralnervensystems führen.

Einen nicht zu übersehenden Faktor stellt die Psyche der schwangeren Frau dar, die durch das unmittelbare Miterleben sämtlicher Manipulationen belastet wird.

Über 95% aller werdenden Mütter ziehen unserer Erfahrung nach der Leitungs-Anaesthesie eine Allgemein-Narkose vor.

Während wir bis zum Jahre 1965 zur Einleitung der Kaiserschnitt-Narkose Thiopental verwendeten, gebrauchen wir seit 1969 ausschließlich Methohexital.

Von der Verwendung des Propanidid sahen wir wegen der beschriebenen Kontraindikationen und der im neueren Schrifttum angeführten Zwischenfälle ab.

Für die Narkose zur Sectio caesarea sollte ein erfahrener Anaesthesist zur Verfügung stehen. Die Patientin ist über alle vorzunehmenden Handlungen aufzuklären. Eine mindestens 6 stündige Nahrungskarenz ist wünschenswert, im Notfall jedoch nicht immer einzuhalten.

Als Prämedikation verabreichen wir routinemäßig 0,5 mg Atropinum sulfuricum und 50 mg Dolatin „Spezial". Wir fanden bei Dolantin-Injektionen, die 30–60 min ante partum gegeben wurden, keine Atemdepressionen des Neugeborenen.

Die Betäubung selbst wird erst nach der Vorbereitung der Schwangeren, also nach Lagerung, Desinfektion der Bauchhaut, Katheterisation und Abdeckung mit sterilen Tüchern eingeleitet.

Auf eine einmalige Gabe von 80–100 mg Methohexital in 1%iger Lösung, die wir langsam injizieren, erfolgen die Injektion von 40 mg Succinylcholin und die intratracheale Intubation. Die Patientin wird so lange mit einem Lachgas-Sauerstoff-Gemisch im Verhältnis von 2:1 beatmet, bis das Kind entwickelt und abgenabelt ist, ein Vorgang, der in unserem Hause 2–5 min in Anspruch nimmt. Die Anaesthesie wird jetzt mit einem Gasgemisch von 25% Sauerstoff und 75% Lachgas fortgesetzt. Zur Narkosevertiefung können wahlweise fraktionierte Methohexital-, Thalamonal- oder Dolantin-Dosen verwendet werden.

Ist eine weitere Relaxierung erforderlich, geben wir intermittierende Mengen von 40 mg Succinylcholin. (Kapfhammer empfiehlt auch für die Mutter nur vorsichtige Dosen, da sich bei Graviden oft ein verminderter

Cholinesterasegehalt des Serums findet, der bei Hepato- und Nephropathien oder Schwangerschaftstoxikosen gefährliche Ausmaße annehmen kann [10]).

Ein Plasmaexpander sollte in jedem Fall schon vor Anaesthesie-Beginn laufen, um einem Volumenmangelschock bei Auftreten einer stärkeren Blutung vorzubeugen.

Die allgemeinen Vorzüge des Methohexitals wurden heute in zahlreichen Vorträgen interpretiert.

Wir stellten zusätzlich fest, daß bei keiner der während der Jahre 1965–1970 mit Methohexital betäubten 151 Mütter während der Anaesthesie Erbrechen oder Aspiration auftrat.

Minimale Methohexitalgaben, optimale Sauerstoff-Sättigung und gute Operationsbedingungen durch ausreichende Muskelerschlaffung verhinderten eine Beeinträchtigung der Neugeborenen.

In APGARS Punktsystem [1], das eine Minute nach der Geburt Herzschlag, Atmung, Muskeltonus, Reflexerregbarkeit und Hautfarbe benotet, erreichten 74% der Kinder die Gesamtziffer 8–10, 19% die Gesamtziffer 6–8. Die verbleibenden 7% entfallen auf Neugeborene mit einer pränatalen Schädigung, auf die die Narkose nur mittelbar Einfluß nahm.

Kardio-vasculäre Depressionen, die bei 5 Müttern auftraten, waren Folge plötzlicher Blutverluste und konnten durch Infusion von Plasmaexpandern bzw. Blut-Transfusionen in kürzester Zeit behoben werden.

Bei der Anaesthesie von Risikofällen mit Schwangerschaftstoxikosen, Eklampsie, Herzfehlern, Stoffwechselerkrankungen, Blutgerinnungsstörungen, Hepato- und Nephropathien, bei denen zudem placentare Funktions- und Durchblutungsstörungen vorliegen, halten wir Methohexital im Gegensatz zu Thiopental für besonders vorteilhaft. Auch im Schockzustand erscheint uns seine Anwendung in reduzierter Dosierung nicht kontraindiziert und relativ gefahrlos.

SLIOM, FRANKEL u. HOLBROCK berichten, daß Methohexital wie alle Barbiturate die Placentarschranke durchschreitet [21]. McKECKNIE u. CONVERSE wiesen schon 1955 nach, daß Thiopental innerhalb von 45 sec im fetalen Blut erscheint und daß nach ca. 3 min äquivalente Blutwerte bei Mutter und Feten gefunden werden [12].

Unsere Untersuchungen mit den in der forensischen Chemie bzw. chemischen Toxikologie üblichen Methoden, die wir wegen Zeitmangels nicht abschließen konnten und über die wir an anderer Stelle berichten, ergaben weder im mütterlichen Venenblut noch im Blut der Nabelschnurvene des Neugeborenen unverändertes Methohexital.

Weitere Versuche, einen Nachweis von Methohexital oder seinen Metaboliten im mütterlichen und kindlichen Blut und Urin durch Gaschromatographie zu erbringen, laufen. (Die Experimente basieren auf der Zusammenarbeit mit Herrn Dr. MAX VON CLARMANN, dem Leiter der Toxikologischen Abteilung des Klinikums rechts der Isar der Technischen Universität München.)

Vollkommene Aufklärung über die Gewebsverteilung von Methohexital und seinen Metaboliten nach dem diaplacentaren Übertritt auf den Fetus könnte nach dem derzeitigen Stand der Forschung nur durch Isotopen erbracht werden. Solange uns diese Methode wegen der möglichen Schädigung des Kindes versagt bleibt, sind wir weiterhin vorwiegend auf klinische Beobachtungen angewiesen.

Zusammenfassung

Die physiologische Disposition der Placenta, des Feten und der Schwangeren stellen besonders hohe und vielfältige Anforderungen an die Allgemein-Anaesthesie für die Sectio caesarea.

Es wird über 151 Kaiserschnitt-Narkosen mit Methohexital in Kombination mit Succinylcholin berichtet.

Individuelle Dosierbarkeit, geringe Toxizität, rasche Elimination bzw. Metabolisierung, minimale zentrale Depression des Kindes und Vermeidung von Hypotension und Erbrechen bei der Mutter lassen uns die Anwendung von Methohexital auch bei Risikofällen besonders vorteilhaft und relativ gefahrlos erscheinen.

Summary

The physiological disposition of the placenta, the foetus, and the pregnant woman make high and manifold demands on the general anaesthesia used for caesarian section.

Our experiences gathered in 151 anaesthesias for caesarian section using methohexital in conjunction with succinylcholine chloride are reported.

The adaptability of the dosage to the needs of the individual case, the low toxicity its rapid elimination and metabolization, the minimum central depression in the child, and the avoiding of vomiting and hypotension in the mother lead us to consider methohexital – even in high-risk cases – to be particularly advantageous and relatively devoid of risk.

Literatur

1. Apgar, V.: Proposal for a new method of evaluation of the newborn infant. Anesth. Analg. Curr. Res. 32, 260 (1953).
2. Beck, L.: Geburtshilfliche Anaesthesie und Analgesie. Georg Thieme Verlag, Stuttgart (1968).
3. Crawford, J. S.: Principles and practice of obstetric anaesthesia. Blackwell, Oxford (1965). Deutsche Übersetzung: Grundlagen und Praxis der geburtshilflichen Anaesthesie. VEB, Verlag Volk und Gesundheit, Berlin (1965).

4. Cugell, D. W., Frank, N. R., Gaensler, E. A., Badger, T. L.: Pulmonary function in pregnancy. Amer. Rev. Tuberc. 67, 568 (1953).
5. Fonts, J. R., Adamson, R. H.: Drug metabolism in the newborn rabbit. Science 129, 897 (1959).
6. Holmes, F.: The supine hypotensive syndrome: its importance to the anaesthetist. Anaesthesia 15, 298 (1966).
7. Howard, B. K.: Shock due to supine hypotensive syndrome. Clin. Obstet. Gynec. 4, 944 (1961).
8. James, L. S.: Physiologic adjustments at birth. Anesthesiology 26, 501 (1965).
9. Jondorf, W. R., Maickel, R. P., Brodie, B. B.: Inability of newborn mice and guinea pigs to metabolise drugs. Biochem. Pharmacol. 1, 352 (1959).
10. Kapfhammer, V.: Muskelrelaxantien in der Geburtshilfe. Z. prakt. Anästh. 1, 360 (1966).
11. Lewis, R. D.: The transference of thiopentone and some relaxants across the placenta. Proc. of the World Congr. of Anesth., Minneapolis, 1955.
12. Mc. Kechnie, F. B., Converse, J. G.: Placental transmission of thiopental. Amer. J. Obstet. Gynec. 70, 639 (1955).
13. Morishima, H. O., Daniel, S. S., Adamson, K., James, L. S.: Effects of positive pressure ventilation of the mother upon the acid-base state of the fetus. Amer. J. Obstet. Gynec. 93, 269 (1965).
14. Motoyama, E. K., Rivard, G., Ackerson, F., Cook, C. D.: Adverse effect of maternal hyperventilation on the fetus. Lancet 1, 286 (1966).
15. Moya, F.: Symposium on obstetrical analgesia and anaesthesia. European Congress of Anaesthesiology. Kopenhagen, Aug. 1966.
16. — Kvisselgard, N.: Placental transmission of succinylcholine. Anesthesiology 22, 1 (1961).
17. — Morishima, H. O., Shnider, S. M., James, L. S.: Influence of maternal hyperventilation on the newborn infant. Amer. J. Obstet. Gynec. 91, 76 (1965).
18. — Smith, E.: Uptake, distribution and placental transport of drugs and anaesthetics. Anesthesiology 26, 465 (1965).
19. Ploman, L., Persson, B. H.: On the transfer of barbiturates to the human foetus and their accumulation in some of its vital organs. J. Obstet. Gynec. Brit. Emp. 64, 706 (1957).
20. Roth, L. J., Barlow, C. F.: Drugs in the brain. Science 134, 22 (1961).
21. Sliom, C. M, Frankel, L., Holbrook, R. A.: A comparison between methohexitone and thiopentone as induction agents for caesarean section anaesthesia. Brit. J. Anaesth. 34, 316 (1962).

Diskussion

Frey: Da einige Redner die Redezeit überschritten haben, sind wir in der Diskussionszeit beschränkt. Ich bitte deshalb, nur noch wichtige Fragen zu stellen. Zunächst hatte sich Herr Whitwam aus London gemeldet.

Whitwam: Ich möchte zunächst auf einen Punkt bezüglich der „Antalgesie" zurückkommen. Die Technik der typischen Kompression wurde erstmals von Clapham u. Brooke eingeführt, dann von Dundee u. Mitarb. popularisiert. Barbiturate senken bei typischen Schmerzreizen die Schmerzschwelle. Robson, Davenport u. Sugiyama wiesen 1965 allerdings nach, daß bei Applikation eines anderen Stimulus, zum Beispiel eines Schmerzreizes an der Haut, also einer Verbrennung Barbiturate gleichzeitig die Schwelle gegenüber typischen Schmerzen senken und die Schwelle gegenüber Hautschmerzen anheben.

Deshalb kann man den Begriff „Antalgesie" nicht so ohne weiteres verwenden. Mit anderen Worten: Schmerzen verschiedenen Ursprungs sind neurologisch verschieden, und das nicht nur im Hinblick auf die moderne Schmerztheorie der „Tor"-Kontrolle, wonach die propriozeptiven Fasern die Fähigkeit haben, das Ausmaß afferenter Impulse des Rückenmarks im Bereich der Hinterwurzel – ausgehend von kleinen sensiblen Fasern, herabzusetzen.

Was die Ausführungen von Kay von heute nachmittag anbelangt, werden Sie mir sicherlich darin zustimmen, daß er, wenn er einen Kältespray auf die Hände der Kinder aufbringt, nicht genügend kühlt, um die Leitung der Nervenfasern in diesen Händen zu blockieren. Im Hinblick auf die „Tor"-Schmerztheorie wird er tatsächlich nichts anderes getan haben, als einen anderen, schmerzlosen Stimulus zu setzen, der den Effekt hat, das spinale „Tor" zu schließen, so daß der schmerzhafte Reiz bei seiner Ankunft nicht so stark empfunden wird. Besten Dank!

Frey: Ich bitte Herrn Schara, der sich als Zweiter zum Wort meldete.

Schara: Nach dem Verlauf der heutigen Tagung, bei der nur Erfreuliches über das Brevimytal berichtet wurde, interessiert mich, wieviel Ampullen-Flaschen Brevimytal bisher verkauft worden sind. Ich frage das deshalb, weil auch vom „Epontol" erst 4 Millionen Ampullen verkauft und entsprechend wenigstens $2^1/_2$ Millionen Narkosen durchgeführt werden mußten, damit über 7 Todesfälle berichtet werden konnte, bei denen ein Zusammenhang mit der Gabe von Epontol nicht von vornherein auszuschließen war.

Ich bin leider in der traurigen Lage, Ihnen über 2 Todesfälle zu berichten, bei denen der Zusammenhang mit Brevimytal zumindest näher geprüft werden müßte.

Im ersten Fall (Abb. 1) traf ein 66jähriger, ungenügend vorbereiteter Mann auf einen eiligen Anaesthesisten. Ich will hier nicht auf die schweren anaesthesiologischen Fehler eingehen, die bei der Behandlung dieses Patienten gemacht worden sind. Mir geht es nur darum, daß, wie aus der Abbildung zu ersehen ist, unmittelbar nach der Injektion von 30 mg Brevimytal zur Narkoseeinleitung der Blutdruck des Patienten unmeßbar wurde und erst nach einer Stunde mittels eines Hypertensin-Tropfes auf meßbare Werte zurückkehrte. Der Patient starb 3 Std nach der Operation auf der Intensiv-Station im Lungenoedem. Die Autopsie ergab eine dekompensierte Hypertonie (Herzgewicht 680 g), alte Infarkte im linken und einen subakuten Infarkt im rechten Herzen.

Sie werden sagen, einen solchen Patienten hätte man mit jedem Narkosemittel umbringen können. Ich bin durchaus Ihrer Meinung und will nur zeigen, daß man es auch mit Brevimytal konnte.

Der zweite Fall betrifft eine 85jährige Frau (Abb. 2), bei der zur Oberschenkelamputation fraktioniert 30 mg (3 × 10 mg) Brevimytal i. v. gegeben wurden. Es kam zu einem kontinuierlichen Abfall des Blutdrucks und nach 20 min zum Herzstillstand. Wiederbelebungsmaßnahmen, die in Anbetracht des Alters und des Allgemeinzustandes der Patientin nur halben Herzens durchgeführt wurden, blieben erfolglos. Auch hier könnte man sagen, es war nicht das Brevimytal, es war das Halothan. Bei dieser Patientin wurde jedoch 4 Wochen früher in Halothan-Narkose mit Ketanest-Einleitung (Abb. 3) ein rupturiertes Aneurysma der Arteria femoralis versorgt. Auch damals kam es zum Blutdruckabfall, jedoch ist zumindest der 2. Abfall durch eine Blutung bedingt gewesen.

Ich will hier nicht behaupten, Brevimytal sei am Tode dieser beiden Patienten schuld. Auf der anderen Seite kann ich aber auch nicht sagen, es habe mit dem Tod dieser beiden Patienten nichts zu tun. Ich kann einen Zusammenhang von vornherein zumindest nicht ausschließen. Ein Zweifel bleibt, und ich meine, daß in der Pharmakologie anders als in der Jurisprudenz im Zweifel nicht für, sondern gegen den Angeklagten entschieden werden muß. Ich möchte also vor der Ansicht warnen, mit Brevimytal gehe man immer sicher. Und wenn hier vorhin jemand, der schon vor 10 Jahren 10% Halothan zur Narkoseeinleitung empfohlen hat, jetzt die Schußeinleitung mit 80–120 mg Brevimytal empfiehlt, dann erweist er uns damit wieder keinen Dienst.

Zindler: Ich habe eine allgemeine Frage, die sich im Grunde genommen wohl jeder stellen muß und hoffe, daß darauf – besonders von unseren ausländischen Referenten – eine Antwort gegeben werden kann. Wir haben – mit Ausnahme der jetzigen Diskussionsbemerkung – immer wieder von

Städt. Krankenanstalten Wuppertal   **Anaesthesie**   D Arzt ☐   Polizei ☐   Strafgefangener ☐   Gutachten ☐

Name: C.B. ♂	Kassenzeichen 51425	Alter: 66	Station:	Datum: 11. 2. 69

Klinische Befunde: (Vorkrankheiten, Laborwerte, EKG)

Asthmat. Emphysembronch.
Exsiccose
abs. Arrhytmie

Blutgr.   Gewicht: Temp.   Hgb: 11,0   Puls   Htkr.   RR 200 110

Gruppe IV:

Diagnose: HAEMATURIE z. B. Blase

Risiko I ☐ II ☐ III ☒ IV ☐ V ☐   Notfall

Praemedikation: DOLANTIN 0,03   ATROPIN 0,0003   Vorabend:

gegeben von: Uhrzeit:

Tageszeit	10 20 30 40 50	8 10 20 30 40 50	9 10 20 30 40 50	10 10 20 30 40 50	Narkosemittel Total: mg, ml, %
Brevimytal		30			30 mg
N₂O		3—1—			l/ min
O₂		1—1—			
Halothan		1——			VOL. %

Narkosemittel

Infusion 220   Plasmaexp. 210   Transfusion 200   Blutverlust 190

○ 500 ml Infusion
● 500 ml Blut
◉ 500 ml Blutersatz

MA.   PL   RH.   BL.   A   A

Anaesth. Technik:

i.v. ☐   i.m. ☐   Maske ☐
Intubation: tracheal ☐   nasal ☐   oral ☒
Tubus   Charr: , mm
Insufflation ☐   nasal ☐   oral ☐
offen ☐   halbgeschl. ☒
halboffen ☐   geschlossen ☐
Atmung: spontan ☐   kontr. ☐   assist. ☒   masch. ☐
Lagerung: Rücken ☒   Bauch ☐   Seite re. ☐   li. ☐
L.A. ☐   P.D. ☐   I.D. ☐
Leit.A. ☐   sacr.Bl. ☐   Plex.Bl. ☐

Anmerkungen:

Blutdruck (V A)   · Puls   X Anaesthesie Beg. u. Ende   ✦ Intub., Ext.   ⊙ Op Beginn u. Ende   Atmung: ○ spontan   A assistiert   K kontrolliert   ~ maschinell.

AKRINOR
SUPRARENIN
NOVADRAL
HYPERTENSIN—TROPF

Anmerkungen:

Postop. Diagnose

Blasenpapillom

Ausgeführte Op.

E.-Resektion — Koagulation

Operateur: Anaesthesist: S.

Zust. d. Pat. beim Verlassen d. Op.
Cornealreflex · ☐   ansprechbar ☐   Kreislauf:
Lidreflex ☐   wach ☐   Atmung:

Postop. Verordnungen: siehe and. Seite ☐

Gruppe V:

54-1-71 F

Abb. 1. Anwendung von 30 mg Methohexital bei der Narkoseeinleitung eines 66jährigen

Städt. Krankenanstalten Wuppertal — Anaesthesie — D Arzt ☐ | Polizei ☐ | Strafgefangener ☐ | Gutachten ☐

Name: J. E. ♀ — Kassenzeichen 57597 — Alter: 85 — Station: — Datum: 18.11.69

Klinische Befunde: (Vorkrankheiten, Laborwerte, EKG) — Blutgr. — Gewicht: 40 kg — Temp. — Hgb. 11,3 — Puls — Gruppe IV: — Htkr. — RR 140/95

Diagnose: Gangrän re. Fuß — Risiko I–V, Notfall — Praemedikation: Atropin 0,00025 — Vorabend: — gegeben von: — Uhrzeit:

Tageszeit: 10 20 30 40 50 | 12 10 20 30 40 50 | 13 10 20 30 40 50 | 10 20 30 40 50 — Narkosemittel Total: mg, ml, %

Narkosemittel:
- Brevimytal — 10 10 10 — 30 mg
- N$_2$O — 3 — l/min
- O$_2$ — 1 — 3 —
- Halothan — 0,7–0,3 — VOL.%
- Succinyl — 20 — 20 mg

Infusion 230 220 — Plasmaexp. 210 — Transfusion 200 — Infusionen Total: ml

Plasmagel

Blutverlust 190 180 170 160 150 140 130 120 110 100

○ 500 ml Infusion
● 500 ml Blut
⊘ 500 ml Blutersatz

Anaesth. Technik:
- I.v. ☐   I.m. ☐   Maske ☐
- Intubation: nasal ☐   tracheal ☐   oral ☒
- Tubus   Charr: mm
- Insufflation ☐   nasal ☐   oral ☐
- offen ☐   halbgeschl. ☒
- halboffen ☐   geschlossen ☐
- Atmung: spontan ☐   kontr. ☒   assist. ☐   masch. ☐
- Lagerung: Rücken ☒   Bauch ☐   Seite re. ☐   li. ☐
- L.A. ☐   P.D. ☐   I.D. ☐   Leit.A. ☐   sacr.Bl. ☐   Plex.Bl. ☐

Blutdruck (V / Λ), · Puls, X Anaesthesie Beg. u. Ende, ◊ Intub., Ext., ⊙ Op Beginn u. Ende, Atmung: ○ spontan, A assistiert, K kontrolliert, ∼ maschinell

90 80 70 60 50 40 30 20 10 0

HERZMASSAGE

O K A A K K K K

Anmerkungen:

X ◊ ⊙

Postop. Diagnose: Gangrän re. Bein

Ausgeführte Op.: O.S. Amputation re.

Operateur: — Anaesthesist: Fe.

Zust. d. Pat. beim Verlassen d. Op.
Cornealreflex ☐   ansprechbar ☐   Kreislauf:
Lidreflex ☐   wach ☐   Atmung: ∅

Postop. Verordnungen: siehe and. Seite ☐ — Gruppe V:

54-1-71 F

Abb. 2. Anwendung von 30 mg Methohexital bei der Narkoseeinleitung einer 85jährigen

Städt. Krankenanstalten Wuppertal   **Anaesthesie**   D Arzt ☐ | Polizei ☐ | Strafgefangener ☐ | Gutachten ☐

Name: J.E. ♀   Kassenzeichen 57597   Alter: 85   Station: Datum: 18.10.69

Klinische Befunde: (Vorkrankheiten, Laborwerte, EKG)   Blutgr.   Gewicht: 40 kg   Temp.

Hgb.   Puls

Gruppe IV: Htkr.   RR

Diagnose: Risiko: I ☐ II ☐ III ☒ IV ☒ V ☐   Notfall ☐   Praemedikation: **Atropin 0,0003**   Vorabend: gegeben von: Uhrzeit:

Tageszeit   10 20 30 40 50   9 10 20 30 40 50 10 10 20 30 40 50 11 10 20 30 40 50   Narkosemittel Total: mg, ml, %

Narkosemittel:
- Ketanest   80   80 mg i.v.
- N₂O   3—2
- O₂   6-1—2   l/min
- Halothan   1-0,5-0,3 —0,5-0,3—   VOL.%
- Succinyl   40   40 mg

Infusion 230 / 220 — ○ G 5   ○ STA.   Infusionen Total: ml ca. 2000 VERLUST

Plasmaexp. 210 — ⊘⊘⊘ Plasmagel

Transfusion 200 — MACRODEX

Blutverlust 190

○ 500 ml Infusion   ● 500 ml Blut   ⊘ 500 ml Blutersatz

180 170 160 150 140 130 120 110 100 90 80 70 60 50 40 30 20 10 0

BLUTUNG

V∧ Blutdruck   · Puls   X Anaesthesie Beg. u. Ende   ◇ Intub., Ext.   ⊙ Op Beginn u. Ende   Atmung: ○ spontan A assistiert K kontrolliert ∿ maschinell

○ ○ K ○ A A A A ○ ○

Anaesth. Technik:
i.v. ☐   i.m. ☐   Maske ☐
Intubation: nasal ☐   tracheal ☐   oral ☒
Tubus   Charr: mm
Insufflation ☐ nasal ☐ oral ☐
offen ☐   halbgeschl. ☒   halboffen ☐   geschlossen ☐
Atmung: spontan ☐ kontr. ☐ assist. ☒ masch. ☐
Lagerung: Rücken ☒ Bauch ☐ Seite re. ☐ li. ☐
L.A. ☐ P.D. ☐ I.D. ☐ Leit.A. ☐ sacr. Bl. ☐ Plex. Bl. ☐

Anmerkungen:

Anmerkungen: X◇ ⊙   ⊙X

Postop. Diagnose   Rupt. Aneurysma Art. femoral. re.

Ausgeführte Op.   Ligatur Art. femoralis re.

Operateur: Anaesthesist: Kr.

Zust. d. Pat. beim Verlassen d. Op.   Cornealreflex ☐   ansprechbar ☐   Kreislauf: Lidreflex ☐   wach ☐   Atmung: Postop. Verordnungen: siehe and. Seite ☐   Gruppe V:

54-1-71 F

Abb. 3. Anwendung von Ketamine und Halothan bei der Narkose der gleichen 85jährigen, die 4 Wochen vorher stattfand

den großen Vorteilen des Methohexital gehört. Man muß sich fragen, warum dieses Mittel, das ja vor 16 Jahren entwickelt wurde und hinsichtlich dessen Stoelting schon 1957 über 25000 Anaesthesien berichtete, sich nicht allgemein durchgesetzt hat. Vielleicht kann einer unserer ausländischen Referenten uns sagen, warum es sich auch in England oder Amerika oder in anderen Bereichen nicht durchsetzte. Im Hinblick auf die heute gehörten großen Vorteile ist das doch eigentlich kaum verständlich.

Coleman: Herr Vorsitzender, ich möchte auf mehrere Punkte zu sprechen kommen. Zunächst einmal zu den beiden mitgeteilten Todesfällen, bei denen Brevimytal eine gewisse Rolle spielte: Wir hörten vorher, daß Brevimytal – und eigentlich jedes intravenöse Narkotikum – bei Patienten mit schwerem Schock und Hypovolämie mit Vorsicht verwendet werden sollte. Dies trifft meines Erachtens für einen oder beide Fälle dieser Diskussionsbemerkung zu. Ich möchte vermuten, daß es wahrscheinlicher eine Fehlverabreichung als irgendein anderer Faktor war.

Was die Zahl der Patienten angeht, die in Großbritannien Brevimytal erhielten, darf ich sagen, daß zumindest ich zu Beginn der 60er Jahre über viele Tausende von Fällen berichtete. Ich weiß weiter, daß meine Kollegen in Derby und in anderen Teilen des Landes das Mittel während der letzten 10 Jahre ständig benutzten.

Auch ich bin der Auffassung, daß das Präparat experimentell wie klinisch gelegentlich in einer Weise benutzt wird, die zu irgendwelchen Komplikationen, besonders zu Singultus, Erbrechen, Muskelbewegungen und Laryngospasmus führen kann.

Es ist in erster Linie ein Hypnoticum, sollte also vorwiegend zur Narkoseeinleitung verwendet werden. Wenn man es zur Fortführung der Anaesthesie anwendet, muß man es mit einem Anaestheticum kombinieren. Ich glaube, daß eine der Ursachen, die dazu beitragen, daß Singultus, Niesen oder diverse Muskelbewegungen ausgelöst werden, darin besteht, daß der operative Eingriff zu früh begonnen wird. Diejenigen von uns, die Brevimytal schon seit Jahren benutzen, wissen sehr gut, daß die vorher festgesetzte Schlafdosis einige Sekunden braucht, um wirksam zu werden. Wenn man eine Störung der Einleitungsphase, also z. B. einen Operationsschmerz zuläßt, entsteht eine Reaktion auf die somatische Stimulierung, die anschließend nur schwer unter Kontrolle zu bringen ist. Dies wurde auch in einem der Vorträge klar zum Ausdruck gebracht.

Langrehr: Ich möchte mich Herrn Schara in der Thematik anschließen. Es ist heute morgen mehrfach gesagt worden, daß bei Zwischenfällen eigentlich viel weniger die verwendeten Substanzen, als vielmehr die durchgeführte Technik immer wieder verantwortlich zu machen ist für das, was passiert. In diesem Zusammenhang möchte ich auf drei Punkte, die heute morgen ganz klar herausgestellt wurden, eingehen. Erstens fand ich es gut, daß Herr Coleman klarstellte, daß man immer mit einer Einleitungsdosis von 1 mg/kg Körpergewicht und weniger auskomme. Auch unserer Erfahrung nach verlangt Methohexital eine individuelle Dosierung. Sie sehen, daß bei einer alten Frau selbst 30 mg schon deletäre Zustände nach sich ziehen können. Man sollte also auch bei dieser Substanz – der Fehler ist oft genug gemacht worden – keine Standarddosierung festlegen.

Der zweite Punkt, eben auch schon angesprochen, ist die „Schußinjektion", die heute morgen zweimal als klar indiziert angegeben wurde. Ich frage mich, ob es überhaupt irgendeinen Grund für eine Schußinjektion von 10 ml der 1%igen Lösung in 10 sec gibt. Auf der anderen Seite kann man, wie die beiden Fälle von Herrn SCHARA zeigen und wie wir bei einer Hypertonikerin gemessen haben, selbst bei langsameren Injektionen 1 min nach der Beendigung der Injektion einen Blutdruckabfall von 210 auf 60 mmHg finden.

Diese Patientin – und damit komme ich zum dritten Punkt – ist vor einem ernsten Zwischenfall ausschließlich dadurch bewahrt worden, daß sie sorgfältigst ventiliert wurde.

Es klang drittens heute morgen immer wieder an, daß man mit Methohexital auch bei fraktionierter Dosierung oder in der Verabreichung durch Infusionen ohne weiteres eine Spontanatmung bestehen lassen könne. Ich dagegen bin der festen Überzeugung, daß dies nicht durchführbar ist, sondern daß man, wenn irgend möglich, die Patienten auch nach Einleitung oder nach fraktionierter Methohexitalgabe assistiert beatmen sollte.

Kay: Eine kurze Antwort an Herrn ZINDLER, der nach der Verwendung des Präparates im Ausland fragte. Wie ich sagte, benutze ich Methohexital, seit es zur Verfügung steht. In meiner Praxis hat es, ebenso wie in den Praxen vieler anderer Ärzte in Großbritannien, Thiopental verdrängt. Was die tatsächlichen Anwendungszahlen angeht, sind diese in der Literatur wohl nicht erfaßt. Meine persönliche Erfahrung bezieht sich auf ungefähr 15- bis 20tausend Fälle.

Frey: Ich danke Ihnen und darf Frau LEHMANN um das Schlußwort bitten.

Schlußwort

Von **Charlotte Lehmann**

Herr Professor FREY, dem ich für die harmonische Zusammenarbeit bei der Vorbereitung und Durchführung des wissenschaftlichen Programmes danken darf, war so liebenwürdig, die Eröffnung der Tagung zu übernehmen und mir das Schlußwort zu überlassen. So sehr ich sonst das „ladies first" begrüße, freue ich mich heute, das letzte Wort behalten zu dürfen.

Schließlich gibt es mir Gelegenheit, der Firma Eli Lilly und Herrn Doktor GMACHL auch in Ihrer aller Namen für die außerordentliche Mühe und Sorgfalt zu danken, die sie für die Arbeiten zur Organisation dieser Tagung verwendeten.

Lassen Sie mich in dem Zusammenhange in aller Offenheit eine Frage ansprechen, die anläßlich solcher Symposien immer wieder gestellt wird. Die Frage nämlich, ob es richtig ist, sich bei einer wissenschaftlichen Tagung der organisatorischen Hilfe und der finanziellen Unterstützung pharmazeutischer und medizinisch-technischer Firmen zu bedienen. Sie stellt sich umso nachdrücklicher, wenn im Mittelpunkt des wissenschaftlichen Meinungs- und praktischen Erfahrungs-Austausches ein Produkt dieser Firma steht.

Verlauf und Ergebnis auch unseres heutigen Symposions sprechen meines Erachtens eindeutig dafür, daß wir diese Frage ohne jeden Vorbehalt bejahen dürfen. Niemand wird daran zweifeln, daß ein Bedürfnis besteht, Tagungen und Symposien hin und wieder einem einzigen Narkosemittel zu widmen. Die Eröterung seiner Indikationsbreite, seiner Vorzüge, seiner Nachteile und seiner spezifischen Risiken führt zwangsläufig zum Vergleich mit anderen Präparaten. Das pharmazeutische Unternehmen, das eine solche Zusammenkunft ermöglicht, fordert diesen Vergleich und damit die kritische Prüfung geradezu heraus.

Keiner, der den Verlauf unserer Arbeitstagungen kennt, wird die Meinung vertreten, Höflichkeit und Dankbarkeit gegenüber der veranstaltenden Firma könnten auf das sachliche Arbeitsergebnis und auf die kritischen Auseinandersetzungen den mindesten Einfluß gewinnen.

Aus meiner eigenen Sicht darf ich sagen, daß ich die Gelegenheit zu einem wissenschaftlich vertieften Erfahrungsaustausch gern wahrnahm, weil wir Methohexital, das wir seit 1962 verwenden und über das wir anhand von Erfahrungen bei mehr als 60 000 Narkosen berichten konnten, schätzen.

Mein besonderer Dank gilt allen den Kolleginnen und Kollegen, die sich der heutigen Tagung als Referenten zur Verfügung stellten oder an der Diskussion beteiligten.

Besonders interessant und wertvoll waren die physiologischen und pharmakologischen Referate, weil sie uns über den tieferliegenden Wirkungsmechanismus des Methohexitals und damit der Narkose überhaupt informierten.

Lassen Sie mich – selbst wenn dies ungewöhnlich erscheinen mag – zum Schluß ein herzliches Wort des Dankes an meine eigenen Mitarbeiter sagen. Trotz der ständigen Arbeitsüberlastung in unserer personell unterbesetzten Abteilung und der relativ kurzen Vorbereitungszeit unterzogen sie sich der Mühe, das uns zur Verfügung stehende, außerordentlich umfangreiche Material zu sichten und erforderliche Untersuchungen anzustellen. Sie trugen durch neun wissenschaftliche Referate zur Klärung wichtiger Fragen über die Anwendungsbreite dieses Narkosemittels bei.

Meine Damen und Herren! Narkosen sind bekanntlich so gut oder schlecht wie der narkoseführende Arzt. Sie gestalten sich in der Hand des Erfahrenen aber umso risikoärmer, je breiter das Spektrum der zur Verfügung stehenden Präparate ist. Uns über eines dieser Mittel noch besser zu informieren, war das Ziel der heutigen Tagung. Ich danke Ihnen allen, daß Sie an diesem Symposium teilnahmen.

Teilnehmerliste

Methohexital – Symposion 5. Dezember 1970

Dr. ANDRES, Selestat
Chef du Département d'Anesthésiologie, Hôpital Civil
Dr. AUBERGER, Hamburg
ChA d. Anästhesie-Abt. d. Frauenklinik Finkenau
Dr. BAUCH, Pforzheim
ChA d. Anästhesie-Abt. am Städt. Krankenhaus
Frau Dr. BAUER-EHNES, München
Anästhesie-Abt. d. Chirurg. Klinik u. Poliklinik d. Klinikums rechts der Isar
Dr. BECKER, Gelsenkirchen
ChA d. Anästhesie-Abt. am Evang. Krankenhaus
Prof. Dr. BEER, München
Institut f. Anästhesiologie d. Chirurg. Univ.-Klinik
Dr. BEHLA, Düsseldorf
ChA d. Anästhesie-Abt. am Allgem. Krankenhaus d. Diakoniewerkes
Dr. BERKEL, Lüdenscheid
ChA d. Anästhesie-Abt. am Städt. Krankenhaus
St.-Medizinalrat Dr. BICKEL, Braunschweig
ChA d. Anästhesie-Abt. d. Städt. Krankenhäuser I u. III
Frau Dr. BIERBRAUER, Heidelberg
Bethanienkrankenhaus
Dr. BOCK, Dortmund
ChA d. Anästhesie-Abt. d. Städt. Krankenanstalten
Dr. BRACK, Oldenburg
Anästhesie-Abt. d. Städt. Krankenanstalten
Frau Dr. BRANDENBURGER, Köln
Anästhesie-Abt. am Evang. Krankenhaus
Dr. BREINL, München
ChA d. Anästhesie-Abt. am Kreiskrankenhaus München-Pasing
Frau Dr. BRENKEN, Münster
Anästhesie-Abt. d. Chirurg. Univ.-Klinik
Dr. BUXTON, London
New Cross Hospital
Dr. BÜCH, Homburg/Saar
Institut f. Pharmakologie u. Toxikologie d. Univ. d. Saarlandes
Frau Dr. BÜCH, Homburg/Saar
OÄ am Institut f. Anästhesie d. Univ.-Kliniken d. Saarlandes
Dr. CANDAS, Essen
OA d. Anästhesie-Abt. d. Krupp-Krankenanstalten
Dr. CARDAN, Münster
Chirurgische Univ.-Klinik
Dr. CHLADEK, Bremen
Anästhesie-Abt. am Zentral-Krankenhaus L. D. W.

Dr. CHRASKA, Bochum
  ChA d. Anästhesie- u. Intensiv-Abt. am Knappschafts-Krankenhaus
Dr. CLEMEN, Heilbronn
  ChA d. Anästhesie-Abt. an d. Städt. Krankenanstalten
Dr. COLEMAN, London
  St. George's Hospital
Dr. COSTA, Remscheid
  Anästhesie-Abt. d. Städt. Krankenanstalten
Frau Dr. DARBOVEN, München
  Anästhesie-Abt. d. Chirurg. Klinik u. Poliklinik rechts der Isar
Prof. EBERLEIN, Berlin
  Dir. d. Instituts f. Anästhesiologie im Klinikum Westend
Dr. EDER, München
  ChA d. Anästhesie-Abt. d. Maria-Theresia-Klinik
Dr. EHRLICHER, Kaiserslautern
  OA d. Zentr. Anästhesie-Abt. am Städt. Krankenhaus
Dr. ELCHLEPP, München
  Anästhesie-Abt. d. Chirurg. Klinik u. Poliklinik rechts der Isar
Dr. ERENGÜL, Krefeld
  OA d. Institut f. Anästhesie- d. Städt. Krankenanstalten
Dr. EULEFELD, Bremerhaven
  ChA d. Anästhesie-Abt. d. Krankenanstalt Wesermünde
Frau Dr. FIEBIG, Heidelberg
  ChÄ d. Anästhesie-Abt. am St.-Josefs-Krankenhaus
Frau Dr. FINK, München
  Anästhesie-Abt. d. Chirurg. Klinik u. Poliklinik rechts d. Isar
Prof. Dr. FREY, Mainz
  Dir. d. Institutes f. Anästhesiologie d. Universität
Dr. FRICK, Itzehoe
  Anästhesie-Abt. d. Städt. Krankenanstalten
Prof. GAUTHIER-LAFAYE, Strasbourg
  Départment d'Anesthésiologie
Dr. GEORGOULIS, Merzig
  ChA d. Anästhesie-Abt. am Kreiskrankenhaus (v. Fellenbergstift)
Dr. GIESECKE, Mainz
Dr. GMACHL, Gießen
  Eli Lilly GmbH
Dr. GRABOW, Gießen
  OA d. Abt. f. Anästhesiologie d. Univ.-Kliniken
Frau Dr. GRAUPNER, Berlin
  Anästhesie-Abt. am Behring Krankenhaus
Dr. GROSS, Köln
  Anästhesie-Abt. am St.-Elisabeth-Krankenhaus
Dr. HARDER, München
  ChA d. Anästhesie-Abt. am Städt. Krankenhaus Schwabing
Dr. HART, Bad-Mergentheim
  Anästhesie-Abt. d. Kreiskrankenhauses
Frau Dr. HARTUNG, München
  Anästhesie-Abt. d. Chirurg. Klinik u. Poliklinik rechts d. Isar
Dr. HEINZE, Bielefeld
  ChA d. Anästhesie-Abt. am St.-Franziskus-Hospital
Prof. Dr. HENNEBERG, Berlin
  OA am Institut f. Anästhesie im Klinikum Steglitz

Dr. Herbst, Frankfurt/M.-Höchst
  ChA am Städt. Krankenhaus, Zentrale Anästhesie-Abt.
Frau Dr. Hlavacek, Frankfurt
  Anästhesie-Abt. am Nordwest-Krankenhaus
Frau Dr. Hofmeister, Stuttgart
  ChÄ d. Anästhesie-Abt. am Marienhospital
Dr. Hostalka, München
  Anästhesie-Abt. d. Chirurg. Univ.-Poliklinik
Prof. Dr. Hutschenreuter, Homburg
  Dir. d. Institutes f. Anästhesie d. Univ.-Kliniken d. Saarlandes
Dr. Jauneau, Strasbourg
  Eli Lilly S. A.
Dr. Junger, Tübingen
  Institut f. Anästhesiologie der Universität
Prof. Dr. Just, Heidelberg
  Dir. d. Institutes f. Anästhesiologie d. Univ.-Kliniken
Frau Dr. Kassner, Unna
  ChÄ d. Anästhesie-Abt. am Evang. Krankenhaus
Dr. Kay, Derby
  Derbyshire Children's Hospital
Dr. Khorssand, Moers
  Anästhesie-Abt. am Krankenhaus Bethanien
Dr. Klaucke, Hamburg
  Anästhesie-Abt. am Bundeswehrlazarett
Dr. Klimpel, Reutlingen
  Anästhesie-Abt. d. Kreiskrankenhäuser Reutlingen u. Urach
Frau Dr. Klimpel, Reutlingen
  Anästhesie-Abt. d. Kreiskrankenhäuser Reutlingen u. Urach
Frau Dr. Krücke, Frankfurt
Frau Dr. Kuhn, Mainz
  Anästhesie-Abt. am St.-Vincenz- u. Elisabeth Hospital
Frau Dr. Kümpers, Münster
  Anästhesie-Abt. an d. Orthopädischen Univ.-Klinik
Dr. Kurka, Coburg
  Anästhesie-Abt. am Landkrankenhaus
Dr. Lamprecht, Berlin
  ChA d. Anästhesie-Abt. am St. Gertrauden-Krankenhaus
Dr. Landauer, München
  Anästhesie-Abt. d. Chirurg. Klinik u. Poliklinik rechts d. Isar
Frau Dr. Landauer, München
  Anästhesie-Abt. d. Chirurg. Klinik u. Poliklinik rechts d. Isar
Dr. Lange, Koblenz
  Anästhesie-Abt. am Zentral-Lazarett d. Bundeswehr
OMR Dr. Langrehr, Bremen-Vegesack
  Dir. d. Allg. Anästhesie-Abt. am Zentralkrankenhaus Bremen Nord
Doz. Dr. Lawin, Hamburg
  ChA d. Anästhesie-Abt. am Allg. Krankenhaus Altona
Frau Dr. Lehmann, München
  ChÄ d. Anästhesie-Abt. d. Chirurg. Klinik u. Poliklinik rechts der Isar
Frau Dr. Lentz, München
  Anästhesie-Abt. d. Univ.-Kinderklinik
Doz. Dr. Lutz, Mannheim
  Dir. d. Anästhesie-Abt. am Klinikum Mannheim d. Univ. Heidelberg

Dr. MANGEL, Bremerhaven
ChA d. Anästhesie-Abt. am Städt. Krankenhaus Mitte
Dr. MANZ, Regensburg
ChA d. Anästhesie-Abt. am Krankenhaus d. Barmherzigen Brüder
Dr. MASCARO, Strasbourg
Département d'Anesthésiologie, Hôpital Civil
Dr. MASSON, Strasbourg
Département d'Anesthésiologie, Hôpital Civil
Frau Dr. MEIER, München
Anästhesie-Abt. d. Chirurg. Klinik u. Poliklinik rechts d. Isar
Dr. MOTTSCHALL, Detmold
ChA d. Anästhesie-Abt. am Kreiskrankenhaus
Frau Dr. MÜNCHHOFF, Frankfurt
OÄ d. Anästhesie-Abt. am St. Katharinen Krankenhaus
Frau Dr. NAGEL, Hannover
OÄ d. Zentralen Anästhesie-Abt. d. Städt. Krankenanstalten
Krankenhaus Siloah
Dr. NEUMANN, Köln
OA d. Anästhesie-Abt. am II. Lehrstuhl d. Chirurgie an der Univ.-Köln im
Städt. Krankenhaus
Dr. NIESEL, Ludwigshafen
ChA d. Anästhesie-Abt. am St.-Marien-Krankenhaus
Doz. Dr. NOLTE, Minden
ChA d. Institutes f. Anästhesiologie d. Zweckverbandes Stadt- u. Kreiskran-
kenhaus
Dr. NÜSSGEN, Hamburg
ChA d. Anästhesie-Abt. am Allg. Krankenhaus Harburg
Prof. OEHMIG, Marburg
Anästhesie-Abt. an d. Chirurg. Univ.-Klinik
Dr. OETTEL, Mainz
Institut f. Anästhesiologie d. Universität
Dr. OPDERBECKE, Nürnberg
ChA d. Anästhesie-Abt. an den Städt. Krankenanstalten
Dr. OSTERKAMP, Frankfurt
ChA d. Anästhesie-Abt. am St.-Katharinen Krankenhaus
Dr. OTT, Nürnberg
ChA d. Anästhesie-Abt. am Krankenhaus Martha-Maria
Frau Dr. PANKOFER-LEPORIS, München
Anästhesie-Abt. am Roten-Kreuz-Krankenhaus I
Frau Dr. PFÄNDER, Bochum
Anästhesie- und Intensiv-Abt. am Knappenschaftskrankenhaus
Frau Dr. PIEPER, Freiburg
ChÄ d. Anästhesie-Abt. am St. Josefs-Krankenhaus
Dr. PLASS, Bremen
Allgem. Anästhesie-Abt. d. Städt. Krankenanstalten
Frau Dr. POHLHAUS, Berlin
Anästhesie-Abt. am Städt. Behringkrankenhaus
Frau Dr. PULPARAMPIL, Hamm
Anästhesie-Abt. am Evang. Krankenhaus
Dr. REDELSTORFF, Recklinghausen
Anästhesie-Abt. am Knappschaftskrankenhaus
Dr. REHFELD, Paris
Eli Lilly S. A.

Frau Dr. Richter, Berlin
ChÄ d. Anästhesie-Abt. am Städt. Krankenhaus Moabit
Frau Dr. Roggenkämper, München
Anästhesie-Abt. d. Chirurg. Klinik u. Poliklinik rechts d. Isar
Frau Dr. Rogowski, Hannover
Krankenhaus Oststadt, Anästh. Zentrum d. Med. Hochschule
Dr. Rudolph, Würzburg
Anästhesiolog. Abt. d. Universität
Dr. Sadisun, Mainz
Dr. Sefrna, Mainz
Institut für Anaesthesiologie
Frau Dr. Siemssen, Pinneberg
Hafenkrankenhaus
Dr. Skarda, Stuttgart
OA d. Anästhesie-Abt. am Katharinen-Hospital
Frau Dr. Soga, München
OÄ am Institut f. Anästhesiologie d. Chirurg. Univ.-Klinik
Dr. Suhayda, Freiburg
Institut f. Anästhesiologie
OMR Dr. Schara, Wuppertal-Barmen
Dir. d. Anästhesie-Abt. d. Städt. Krankenanstalten
Frau Dr. Schäfer, Augsburg
ChÄ d. Anästhesie-Abt. d. Städt. Kliniken
Dr. Schlaak, Neuss
ChA d. Anästhesie-Abt. d. Lukas-Krankenhauses
Dr. Schlagintweit, München
Anästhesie-Abt. am Städt. Krankenhaus Harlaching
Frl. Dr. Schmitz, Lübeck
Anästhesie-Abt. d. Medizinischen Akademie
Dr. Schottky, Bochum
OA d. Zentr. Anästhesie-Abt. d. Berufsgenossenschaftlichen Krankenanstalten
„Bergmannsheil"
Dr. Schüler, Berlin
Städt. Klinik f. Lungenkranke Heckeshorn
Dr. Schulte-Vels, Freiburg
Institut f. Anästhesiologie d. Kliniken d. Universität
Dr. Schwiete, Bochum
Anästhesie-Abt. am St.-Josefs-Hospital
Dr. Stanek, Gießen
Eli Lilly GmbH
Doz. Dr. Stöcker, Essen
Anästhesie-Abt. am Klinikum Essen der Ruhr Universität
Prof. Dr. Stoffregen, Göttingen
Anästhesie-Abt. d. Göttinger Univ.-Kliniken
Doz. Dr. Stolz, Tübingen
OA d. Institutes f. Anästhesiologie d. Universität
Dr. Strubelj, Bottrop
Anästhesie-Abt. am Knappschaftskrankenhaus
Frau Dr. Stümper, Wuppertal-Elberfeld
ChÄ d. Anästhesie-Abt. an den Städt. Ferdinand-Sauerbruch-Kranken-
anstalten
Dr. Tatai, Hannover
Zentrale Anästhesie-Abt. d. Städt. Krankenanstalten Krankenhaus Siloah

Dr. Thiemens, Ulm
   Abt. für Anästhesiologie der Universität
Dr. Tümer, Hildesheim
   OA d. Anästhesie-Abt. d. Städt. Krankenhauses
Dr. Warncke, Bremerhaven
   ChA d. Anästhesie-Abt. am St.-Joseph-Hospital
Doz. Dr. Wawersik, Heidelberg
   OA d. Abt. f. Anästhesiologie d. Chirurg. Univ.-Klinik
Dr. Weber, Köln
   ChA d. Anästhesie-Abt. am Elisabeth-Krankenhaus
Dr. Wehrschütz, Gießen
   Eli Lilly GmbH
Dr. Weigand, Köln
   Anästhesie-Abt. an der HNO-Klinik d. Universität
Dr. Weimann, Hannover
   Anästhesie-Abt. am Friederikenstift
Prof. Dr. Weis, Würzburg
   Anästhesie-Abt. d. Universität
Dr. Wessely, München
   Anästhesie-Abt. d. Orthopädischen Klinik
Dr. Whitwam, London
   Hammersmith Hospital
Frau Dr. Wilckens, München
   Anästhesie-Abt. d. Chirurg. Klinik u. Poliklinik rechts d. Isar
Dr. Wunsch, Dortmund
   ChA d. Anästhesie-Abt. am Knappschaftskrankenhaus
Dr. Zierl, München
   ChA d. Anästhesie-Abt. am Krankenhaus d. Dritten Ordens

Anaesthesiology and Resuscitation · Anaesthesiologie und Wiederbelebung
Anesthésiologie et Réanimation